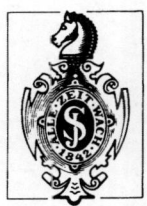

Treatment in Clinical Medicine

Series Editor: John L. Reid

Hilary A. Capell · T.J. Daymond
W. Carson Dick

Rheumatic Disease

Springer-Verlag
Berlin Heidelberg New York Tokyo 1983

Hilary A. Capell, MRCP
Consultant Physician, Centre for Rheumatic Diseases,
Baird Street, Glasgow, Scotland

T.J. Daymond, MRCP, DPhys Med
Consultant Rheumatologist, Sunderland District General
Hospital, Sunderland, England

W. Carson Dick, MD, FRCP
Reader in Rheumatology, University of Newcastle upon Tyne,
Consultant Rheumatologist, Royal Victoria Infirmary,
Newcastle upon Tyne, England.

Series Editor:
John L. Reid, MD, FRCP
Regius Professor of Materia Medica,
University of Glasgow, Scotland

ISBN-13:978-3-540-12622-5   e-ISBN-13:978-1-4471-3113-7
DOI: 10.1007/978-1-4471-3113-7

Library of Congress Cataloging in Publication Data
Capell, H. (Hilary), 1949-
Rheumatic Disease (Treatment in Clinical Medicine)
Includes bibliographies and index. 1. Rheumatism—Addresses, essays, lectures. I.
Daymond, T. (Terence), 1942-   . II. Dick, W. Carson (William Carson), MD.
III. Title. IV. Series. [DNLM: 1. Arthritis—Drug therapy. 2. Arthritis—Therapy.
WE 344 C238r] RC927.C325 1983 616.7′23   83-12398
ISBN-13:978-3-540-12622-5(U.S.)

Typeset by Wilmaset, Birkenhead, Merseyside

2128/3916-543210

Series Editor's Foreword

"Rheumatic Disease" is the second monograph in a new series on management and treatment in major clinical subspecialties and patient groups. Further volumes will be published over the next few years. Each book is complete in its own right. The whole series, however, has been prepared to fill a gap, perceived by the publisher, myself and the volume authors, between standard textbooks of medicine and therapeutics and research reviews, symposia and original articles in specialist fields. Each volume aims to provide a concise, up to date account of treatment in its subject area with particular reference to drug therapy. Wherever possible, authorship has been undertaken by practising clinicians who themselves have training and experience in clinical pharmacology. The volumes are intended to be guides to treatment, to assist in the choice of drug and other treatment and to provide easy references to drug interactions and adverse reactions.

The aims of the series should be upheld by this volume on "Rheumatic Disease". The book has been prepared in Glasgow and Newcastle. The authors, Drs. Hilary Capell, Terry Daymond and Carson Dick, are not only respected clinicians and rheumatologists but have wide clinical and research experience in the clinical pharmacology of antirheumatic drugs and therapeutic management of connective tissue disease and other areas of rheumatology. This volume combines practical pragmatic management with new concepts in drug treatment. Rheumatic diseases are reviewed in the first 12 chapters from a pathophysiological viewpoint. Clinical problem areas such as neck pain, back pain and shoulder pain are given prominence along with well recognised disease entities such as gout and rheumatoid arthritis. Rheumatic complications of systemic diseases are also included.

In the second part of the volume, principles of management are considered and drug therapy is presented in perspective. There are detailed descriptions of the clinical pharmacology, use and adverse reactions occurring with major classes of drugs used in rheumatology, including non-steroidal anti-inflammatory drugs, steroids and other second line therapy.

This volume follows the first volume in the Series on "Gastro-intestinal Disease". Subsequent volumes will include "The Elder-ly" by W. MacLennan, A. Shepherd and I.H. Stevenson, Cardiovascular Disease, Respiratory Disease, Neurological and Neuro-psychiatric Disorders, and Hypertension.

Glasgow, July 1983   John L. Reid

Preface

As our knowledge of acute diseases has increased and our ability to treat them has improved, so the relative importance of chronic disease and disability has become more clamant. The past 50 years have seen a dramatic change in our attitude to the chronic rheumatic diseases in particular. We have progressed rapidly from an attitude of aspirin, splinting and despair or even rejection to the present position where we have new drugs, new operations and, most important of all, a new understanding of the underlying mechanisms responsible for these diseases. It hardly needs to be stressed that patients with arthritis present an immense challenge to the developed countries, particularly in terms of morbidity. Rheumatic disorders today account for one-seventh of all morbidity and one-half of disability beyond the age of retirement in the United Kingdom. The amount of money lost to the revenue of this country as a result of arthritis and rheumatism exceeds by far that lost due to industrial action (Office of Health Economics 1977; Wood 1977). The cost to the individual in terms of pain and suffering cannot be computed so easily.

The advances in this subject have occurred against the backcloth of the scientific, technological and therapeutic revolution of the past 40 years which, despite the arguments of Ivan Illich and Bernard Dixon, has transformed the lives of countless patients throughout the world. However, this has not been achieved without cost. Iatrogenesis, in many cases avoidable, has become increasingly frequent. It is therefore of major importance to be aware of the therapeutic ratio, the ratio between the efficacy of a compound and its adverse reactions. In this book we present a rational and simple approach to the management of patients suffering from rheumatic diseases. The emphasis of the text is upon management and we have therefore included only a concise summary of the aetiology, pathogenesis and clinical features of the various diseases. There is an abundance of other sources to which we refer the reader for further details on these topics.

One of the greatest challenges to confront a clinician is the management of a patient with one of the rheumatic diseases. Treatment must be planned over years or even decades, precluding prescription of temporarily effective remedies with prohibitive long-term toxicity such as corticosteroids except in a limited number of very clearly defined circumstances. The doctrine of *primum non nocere* is fundamental to the practise of sound rheumatology.

References

Office of Health Economics (1977) Physical impairment; social handicap. ISSN 0473 8837 (No. 60)
Wood PNH (ed) (1977) The challenge of arthritis and rheumatism. Available from: The British League Against Rheumatism, c/o The Arthritis and Rheumatism Council, 41 Eagle St., London WC1R 4AR

Further Reading

In accordance with the focus of this text we have listed at the end of each section suggestions for further reading. In some of the sections, in particular those dealing with drug treatment, these are more detailed than in other sections where they are more in the nature of review material. We have tried to provide references suitable for individuals with a very wide spectrum of interest.

The most important sources of further reading are the following large textbooks of rheumatology:

Corrigan B, Maitland GD (1983) Practical orthopaedic medicine, 1st edn. Butterworths, London
Goodman WS, Gillman AC (eds) (1980) The pharmacological basis of therapeutics, 6th edn. Macmillan, New York
Hollander JL, McCarty DJ Jr (eds) (1979) Arthritis and allied conditions, 9th edn. Lea and Febiger, Philadelphia
Kelly W, Harris ED Jr, Ruddy S, Sledge CB (eds) (1981) Textbook of rheumatology, 1st edn. Saunders, Philadelphia London Toronto
Scott JT (ed) (1978) Copeman's textbook of the rheumatic diseases, 5th edn. Churchill Livingstone, Edinburgh London New York

In addition the following texts are available to amplify various sections of this text:

Bird HA, Wright V (1979) Applied drug therapy of the rheumatic diseases. Wright-PSG, Bristol London Boston
Dick WC (1981) Immunological aspects of rheumatology. MTP Press, Lancaster

Dick WC, Moll JMH (1983) Recent advances in rheumatology, 3rd edn. Churchill
    Livingstone, Edinburgh London New York
Feinstein AR (1977) Clinical biostatistics. Mosby, Saint Louis
Hart FD (ed) (1981) Drug treatment of the rheumatic disease, 2nd edn. Adis Health
    Science Press, Sydney
Katz WA (1977) Rheumatic diseases; diagnosis and management. Lippincott,
    Philadelphia Toronto
Maini RN, Berry H (1981) Modulation of autoimmunity and disease; the
    penicillamine experience. Praeger Special Studies, Praeger Scientific, New
    York
Resnick D, Niwayama G (1981) Diagnosis of bone and joint disorders. Saunders,
    Philadelphia London Toronto

Contents

1 Introduction

Arthritis is an emotive word, vulnerable to the mass media and to folklore. Patients use words like "arthritis", "rheumatism" and "fibrositis" in a context which is unfamiliar to the physician, and conversely, much of the doctor's vocabulary might as well be a foreign language for all it conveys to the patient. The doctor's first task is to establish common ground with the patient and it is at this stage that it is so important for a doctor to have a wide experience of art, religion, literature, the local culture and the lifestyle of the patient before him. How can a clinician expect to find common ground with a patient whose philosophy, religion or day-to-day activities are a closed book to him? This is a matter of particular importance in rheumatology, where a major determinant of the therapeutic outcome is the relationship between the doctor and the patient. Indeed, it is likely that this is of more importance than the selection of any particular drug therapy.

It is impossible to overemphasise the importance of the clinical history. Separate consideration should be accorded to each of the patient's complaints. This is the teaching of the eleventh century Middle Eastern physician Avicenna (Ibnecenna) and it finds particular relevance in rheumatology. By listening to the patient without prejudice he was able to recognise more than 15 distinct and separable pain syndromes. The pain associated with the acute flitting non-destructive arthritis of rheumatic fever is different from the pain associated with an exacerbation of proliferative destructive rheumatoid arthritis and this may be apparent to the patient afflicted by both diseases.

As the symptom of pain is so important, being the primary cause of referral in the majority of instances, it is worth taking time to define it clearly. Time and circumstances surrounding onset, evolution, remission and exacerbation, site and radiation, and other associated features must be recorded and severity may be expressed upon a numerical or adjectival scale using the English adjectives of degree. Precise localisation of the site of maximal pain or tenderness in a peripheral joint yields information of fundamental importance (Fig. 1.1) and assists diagnosis more than any laboratory test. The common trap of failing to recognise that pain is often referred to the joint distal to the one affected should be remembered. Pain felt entirely within the knee may mark the presence of

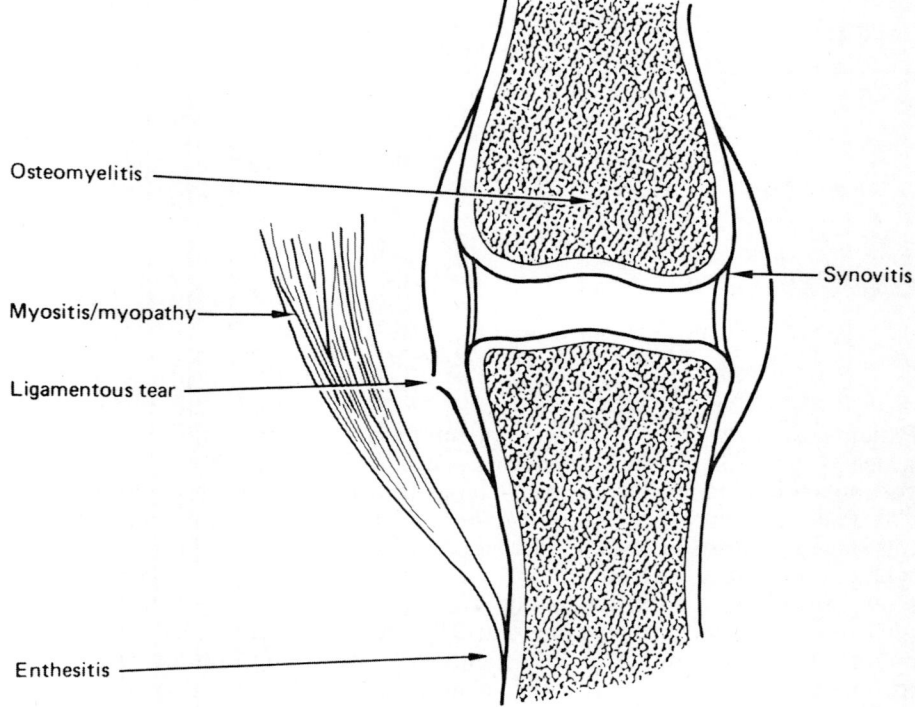

Osteomyelitis

Myositis/myopathy

Ligamentous tear

Enthesitis

Synovitis

Fig. 1.1. Precise localisation of the site of maximal tenderness

disease confined to the hip joint and be due to radiation down the obturator nerve, while pain in the region of the hip may originate from disease of the lumbar spine. Similarly, in the upper limb pain experienced in the region of the shoulder may be produced by radiation, the site of the offending pathology being the cervical spine.

A useful clue may be afforded by the plane or planes of movement which are associated with the production of pain. Pain produced both by active and by passive movement in all planes marks the affected site as being intra-articular or closely associated with the joint capsule. Pain in the lumbar spine, for example, may be present in only one plane. Pain on flexion alone may indicate a disc lesion whereas pain on extension is the hallmark of a disorder of the facet joint. Pain elicited by a particular movement may indicate a lesion of the relevant muscle, tendon, ligament or enthesis subserving that movement. The enthesis is the site of insertion of a muscle through tendon or ligament into bone. Inflammatory lesions commonly produce pain in more than one direction of both active and passive movement and pain is then associated with stiffness.

The second major symptom of which a patient may complain is stiffness. It is very important to elicit this symptom separately from pain and to be certain that the patient understands the distinction. It is the symptom of stiffness which is characteristically worse in the morning and after resting ("gelling") in the inflammatory arthritides. When pain in the back is associated with pronounced stiffness this directs attention to the presence of one of the inflammatory spondarthritides whereas in the absence of stiffness diagnosis is more likely to be structural or mechanical in nature. Stiffness may be quantitated in terms of both severity and duration and again the English adjectives of degree usually suffice and are most easily understood by the patient.

The next symptom which gives the most useful information is loss of function. It is sad to record that although this is of fundamental importance to the patient, it is nevertheless a symptom which physicians find very difficult to record quantitatively in a sensible manner. Functional indices which provide useful information sensitively are often too time consuming for routine use and the more convenient and simpler indices are often too insensitive to record small but significant changes.

The importance of functional disability is emphasised by the fact that reconstructive surgery is carried out to improve function, not for cosmetic reasons (Chap. 20). It is very important to assess function in detail. The tasks which the patient finds difficult should be discussed separately and should be dissected. It is striking that our view of physical disability is still influenced considerably by the 1939–1945 war. Even the forms which we have to complete are oriented to static disability such as loss of a limb. However, far more often we are faced with a patient with fluctuating problems who can perform a task with ease one day yet finds it impossible to complete that same task a day later or even at a different time on that same day. Wherever possible, functional assessment should be conducted as close to the patient's home and work environment as possible.

Other symptoms which yield useful information include a feeling of exhaustion and inability to complete simple tasks, which is a frequent early symptom in inflammatory arthritides such as rheumatoid arthritis, and depression. Again, the word depression demands subclassification (Chap. 8). The fear of losing independence is a very major feature even if it is not volunteered to the physician.

The clinical signs which are of most value are tenderness, which is closely intercorrelated with pain, and the presence of swelling. As with pain, it is very important to determine the site of maximal tenderness precisely (Fig. 1.1). If swelling is present it is necessary to distinguish whether it is due to soft tissue involvement or to bony enlargement. If the swelling is soft tissue in nature then it is important to distinguish between a synovial effusion, synovial hypertrophy and extra-articular swelling.

Each patient who is suffering from a chronic arthritis should be documented thoroughly and one of the most simple methods of achieving this is to construct in graph form the evolution of the disease. Examples of this are shown in Figs. 1.2 and 1.3. A simple severity scale, again based upon the English adjectives of degree, serves for the vertical axis and the horizontal axis must be designed to cope on the one hand with day-to-day variation during phases of increased activity or during times of therapeutic decision and on the other with year-to-year variation throughout inactive phases.

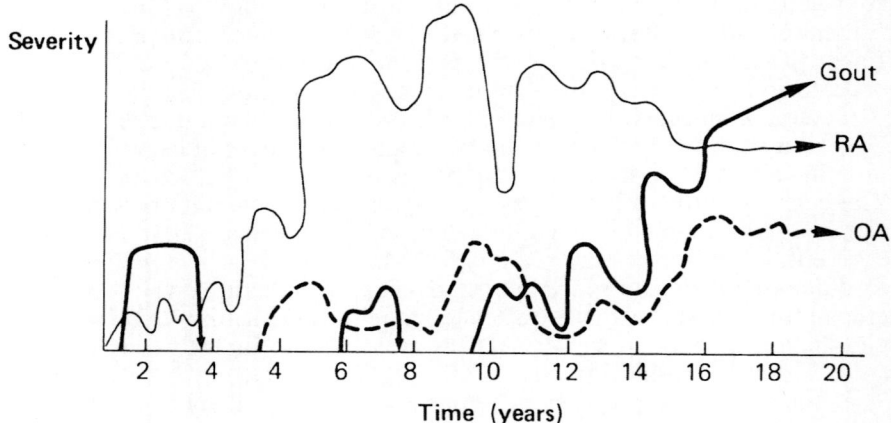

Fig. 1.2. Evolution of different types of chronic arthritis. Note that in gout the joint may return to complete normality between attacks, this being rare in diseases such as rheumatoid arthritis. *RA*, rheumatoid arthritis; *OA*, osteoarthritis

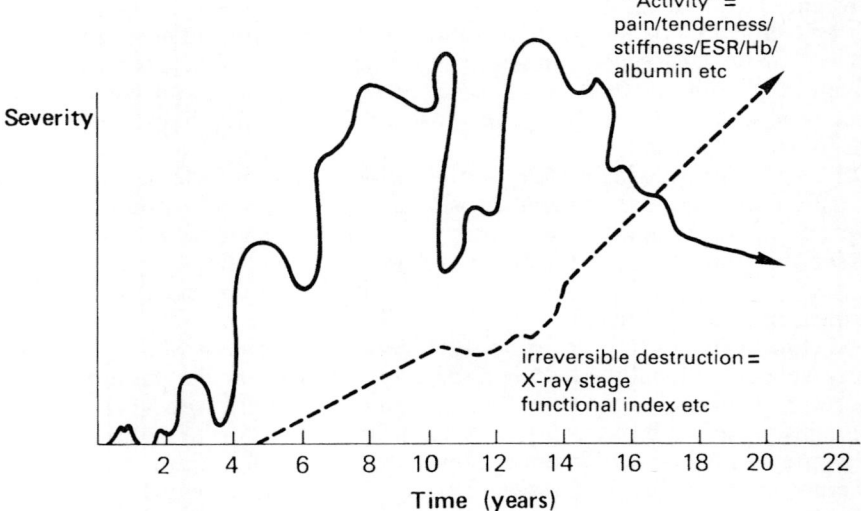

Fig. 1.3. Evolution of arthritis in a patient with rheumatoid arthritis. Note that the decision when to consider surgical intervention is less arbitrary when such graphic information is available. The therapeutic goal which is becoming more and more clamant is the progressive irreversible destruction in, for example, a surgically accessible joint such as the hip. Here it becomes obvious that consultation with the surgeon is required. (See p. 72 for full discussion.)

The construction of such a graph takes very little time and is of considerable assistance at times when therapeutic decisions must be taken. If disease activity is plotted in one colour and the component of the disease which represents irreversible underlying deformity (mirrored for example in rheumatoid arthritis by the X-ray stage and the functional index) in another, then decisions such as when to consider surgical intervention become less arbitrary.

The importance of the clinical history and examination cannot be overemphasised. If it is not possible to form a diagnosis after a well-taken history and thorough clinical examination then it is unlikely to become easier later. Ninety per cent of rheumatology is encompassed by the history and clinical examination allied with compassion and common sense. Hence our emphasis upon precision is not disproportionate.

The rheumatologist could well take a leaf from the book of the psychiatrist where greater stress is laid upon the full description, or "formulation", of the *person* before the *patient* before the *disease*. Thus instead of the diagnosis or pseudodiagnosis "rheumatoid arthritis" we should be recording "a chronic painful progressive destructive nodular and inflammatory disease of peripheral joints distributed in a symmetrical manner, complicated by anaemia and reactive depression, and occurring in the setting of a previously fit young married female with a high morale and a well-developed sense of humour."

2 General Principles and Approach to the Patient in the Context of Osteoarthritis

Introduction

Osteoarthritis has a venerable history, having been recorded in Egyptian mummies and in dinosaurs of the Pleistocene era. It is now obvious that the term osteoarthritis represents a syndrome, not a disease. Furthermore the term means different things to different people. To the pathologist it implies fibrillation and destruction of the cartilage surface with clustering of chondrocytes around the bases of deep clefts, remodelling and sclerosis of subchondral bone, changes in the composition and characteristics of synovial fluid and the development of marginal osteophytes. To the radiologist the word suggests loss of joint "space" (reflecting cartilage destruction), osteophytosis, bone cysts and increased density of subchondral bone. To the clinician the word conjures up a picture of a very common clinical problem where the patient complains of pain more than stiffness, and of functional disability but where the disease process is confined essentially to one or to a few affected joints.

Cellular Basis of the Disease

The principal tissue affected is cartilage but changes occur in all joint structures. Cartilage consists of cells (chondrocytes) lying in a matrix which they themselves produce. Interwoven in this matrix are collagen fibres which provide great tensile strength, between which are trapped the globular macromolecular proteoglycans which confer elasticity and resistance to deformation. Recently there has been an explosion in knowledge of the molecular basis of a multiplicity of diseases which affect primarily collagen (Table 2.1) or proteoglycan (Table 2.2), these being legitimate contenders for the description "connective tissue diseases".

Table 2.1. Conditions associated with molecular defects in collagen. OA, osteoarthritis; E-D, Ehlers-Danlos; PSS, progressive systemic sclerosis; RA, rheumatoid arthritis

Nature of defect	Clinical condition
Collagen chain synthesis	E-D 4, Osteogen.Imp. ? OA
Hydroxyproline syntheses	Scurvy
Hyroxylysine synthesis	E-D 4
Procollagen–collagen conversion	E-D 7
Oxidative deamination of (OH) lysine	E-D 5, Menke's kinky hair syndrome, cutis laxa
Crosslink formation	Homocystinuria, Marfan's syndrome, D-penicillamine
Increased rate of collagen synthesis	PSS, keloid, cirrhosis pulmonary fibrosis
Decreased rate of collagen synthesis	Corticosteroids, ageing, osteopaenia
Increased rate of collagen degradation	RA, hormonal effects
Decreased rate of collagen degradation	Some cases of scleroderma/PSS

Table 2.2. Lysosomal storage diseases

Disorder	Enzyme defect
1. *Mucopolysaccharidoses* (MPS)	
MPS1	α-L-iduronidase
MPS 2	Iduronate sulphatase
MPS 3	
a) Sanfillipo A	Heparan-N-sulphatase
b) Sanfillipo B	N-ac-α-glucosaminidase
c) Sanfillipo C	Ac-Co-A:α-glucosamine-N-acetyl-transferase
MPS 4	N-Ac-galactosamine-6-sulphatase
MPS 6	N-Ac-galactosamine-4-sulphatase
MPS 7	β-glucuronidase
MPS 8	N-Ac-glucosamine-6-sulphatase
2. *Mucolipidosis* (ML)	
ML 1	Acid neuraminidase
ML 2 (I-cell disease)	?
ML 3 (pseudo-Hurler polydystrophy)	?
ML 4	?
Unclassified	
3. *Glycoproteinoses*	
Mannosidosis	α-mannosidase
Fucosidosis	α-fucosidase
Aspartylglucosaminuria	Aspartylglucosamine aminohydrolase
4. *Gangliosidoses*	
GM1	
a) Generalised gangliosidosis	β-galactosidase ABC
b) Juvenile gangliosidosis	β-galactosidase BC
c) O-galactosidase variant	β-galactosidase
GM 2 (Sandhoff disease)	Hexosaminidase A and B
5. *Others*	
Metachromatic leucodystrophy	Multiple sulphatases
Farber's disease	Ceraminidase
Geleophysic dwarfism	?

Cartilage is avascular; thus chondrocytes depend upon diffusion from subchondral bone vessels and from synovial fluid for metabolic exchange. There is a low turnover of these cells and their metabolic products in vivo, although if chondrocytes are removed from that environment they demonstrate a normal cell turnover time in vitro. This suggests that it is something in their own matrix which is inhibiting them from dividing and synthesising at a faster rate in vivo.

The function of cartilage is to provide a smooth surface allowing moving parts of the skeleton to glide over one another. Movement of a joint is also dependent upon all other structures, including joint capsule, ligaments, tendons and surrounding muscles, as well as the congruity of the bony articulating surfaces. For example, the intricate internal mechanism of the knee joint with its internal cruciate ligaments and menisci allows a degree of rotation in constrained directions in addition to flexion and extension. The stability of this joint is dependent upon the strength of its surrounding ligaments, tendons and muscles rather than the congruity of the articulating surfaces. The opposite is true in the case of the hip joint. In this instance the congruity of the articulating surfaces is the primary factor in the stability of the joint. The shoulder is almost unique in its requirement for the maximum range of movement in all planes, and it depends for stability upon its surrounding powerful muscles and tendons. In contrast, the primary function of the lower lumbar spine is to resist deformation, and again anatomy subserves function. The central spinal joints have no synovial lining, i.e. they are not diarthrodial joints. When diseases such as rheumatoid arthritis or osteoarthritis afflict the spine then it is the synovial lined apophyseal joints which are involved most prominently. Involvement of the central spinal joints is termed degenerative disc disease, which very often coexists with osteoarthritis of the spinal diarthrodial apophyseal joints, both becoming more common with advancing years. The disc with its nucleus pulposus and powerful concentric rings of annulus fibrosus is ideally suited to its central purpose of resistance to deformation.

An area of vital importance to our understanding of normal and diseased joint function which has undergone a transformation in recent years is biomechanics. Synovial fluid—an ultrafiltrate of plasma plus secretions from the synovial lining cells, including proteoglycan—is present in small amounts in all diarthrodial joints. It provides a contribution to joint lubrication. Synovial fluid in normal persons is viscous and exhibits non-Newtonian properties which are lost in various disease states. Similarly, the constituents of synovial fluid change considerably in disease, and in particular the fluid in inflammatory joint diseases reflects the underlying inflammatory and immunological events. Cells, low molecular weight mediators of inflammation and potentially destructive acidic and neutral high molecular weight proteinases accumulate and may contribute to the perpetuation, if not to the initiation, of the pathological processes. The main arguments against these synovial constituents as prime movers in tissue destruction rest upon the patchy as opposed to discrete early lesions and the fact that the enzymes are present in inhibitor excess. It is becoming more and more likely that the site of action of these enzymes is pericellular.

The study of the biomechanical properties of synovial fluid and of other joint constituents is a recent phenomenon and owes much to the stimulus provided by one of the most exciting advances in medicine of the past decade, namely the success of artificial joint replacement. Similarly, it is only recently that attention has been focussed upon the state of the underlying bone. Cartilage is a poor shock absorber, and since all joints are subjected to repetitive irregular impulse loading, the forces generated must be absorbed by surrounding soft tissue and especially bone. In this regard the state of the underlying subchondral bone is of considerable importance. It has been suggested that abnormal stiffness of that bone is an early, if not a primary finding, in osteoarthritis. It is possible that this may explain the protection afforded to the joint by osteoporosis, in which the underlying bone is softer, more easily deformed and better able to absorb forces than normal bone. It is certainly true that osteoarthritis rarely coexists with osteoporosis. Biomechanics has already given us much information and it is likely that we are seeing only the beginning of a burgeoning new subject.

Aetiopathogenetic Considerations

The development of osteoarthritis depends upon a combination of biophysical and biochemical changes acting within the cartilage. Ageing alone is a necessary but not a sufficient cause for the development of osteoarthritis. Not all joints within the same individual demonstrate the same degree of osteoarthritis and, conversely, a proportion of individuals in their second decade suffer from this process. Age-related changes, including changes in matrix composition and pigmentation, may be recognised distinct from osteoarthritis. Ageing, however, may permit other mechanisms time to exert their individual effect and time for that effect to become manifest. Certainly any process which alters the congruity of the articulating surfaces leaves that joint with an enhanced risk of the subsequent development of osteoarthritis and this is the explanation of the large number of different circumstances which are associated with the development of so-called secondary osteoarthritis (Table 2.3). Whether or not there is such a distinct entity as "primary" osteoarthritis is more difficult to discern. This description may be simply an expression of our present ignorance in that we have not yet recognised the underlying secondary cause in that instance. For example, it has been suggested that many patients labelled as having primary osteoarthritis of the hip in fact owe the genesis of their disease to an unrecognised minor congenital anomaly. On the other hand we have the example of rickets to caution us. In that instance it was only after all the secondary environmental factors were removed that it became possible to recognise the existence of a distinct small subgroup who were suffering from a genetically determined inborn error of metabolism.

Table 2.3. Classification of "secondary osteoarthritis"

Congenital/developmental	Hip dysplasias, shallow acetabulum, slipped epiphysis, femoral neck abnormalities, multiple epiphyseal dysplasia, osteochondritis, Morquio's syndrome, Perthes' disease, primary protrusio
Traumatic	Acute
	Chronic (industrial/sport etc.)
	Charcot's joint
Inflammatory	All of the inflammatory arthritides
Endocrine	Acromegaly, diabetes, hypothyroidism, primary and iatrogenic Cushing's syndrome
	Abnormalities of sex hormones
Metabolic	Gout, haemochromatosis, haemophilia, ochronosis, calcium pyrophosphate crystal deposition disease, Paget's disease, and all above inborn errors of metabolism (Tables 2.1 and 2.2.)

However osteoarthritis is initiated, there is evidence of a final common path leading to further tissue destruction and clinical disease. Fibrillation and destruction of cartilage, accompanying fluctuating inflammatory synovitis and changes in subchondral bone are countered by nature's attempt at healing. The early clustering of chondrocytes around the fibrillating clefts probably represents a tissue reaction to the initial process but there is evidence that the collagen and proteoglycan which these cells are producing are themselves abnormal. Similarly, the development of osteophytes from the joint margin may be reactive and may be an attempt to mitigate further damage by increasing the effective load-bearing area. In the hip which is the seat of exuberant osteophytosis, cartilage loss is least and in such joints cartilage regeneration measured by increase in radiological joint "space" has been documented. However, it is equally obvious that these very osteophytes either by their physical presence or by breaking off into the joint cavity may produce clinical symptoms in their own right. The synovial tissue may be inflamed and this may produce fluctuating symptoms quite distinct from the underlying process and may benefit from treatment. In the later stages the synovium is often remarkably acellular and fibrosed.

Osteoarthritis and degenerative disc disease often coexist and in the spine both may produce an identical clinical picture. The term "spondylosis" is used to express a combination of symptoms and signs which may be produced by either or both. The process in degenerative disc disease is similar in many ways to that in osteoarthritis but there is no element of synovitis. There is disruption and destruction of collagen fibres and matrix proteoglycan and protrusion may occur either vertically through the vertebral plate or horizontally. In the latter a midline protrusion, although by far the least likely, is the most dangerous since it so often involves the spinal cord or cauda equina. This is a surgical emergency. More commonly protrusion occurs in a posterolateral direction producing characteristic signs and symptoms locally and through involvement of the emerging nerve roots. In the cervical spine the additional element of the closely related vertebral arteries must be remembered, and both disc disease and osteophytosis may encroach upon these blood vessels, producing symptoms and signs due to vascular insufficiency.

The clinical presentation of patients with disease in the central joints is outlined in Chap. 3. The remainder of this chapter is devoted to the clinical features and management of patients with osteoarthritis of the peripheral joints.

Clinical Features

Pain is the most important and usually the first symptom. Initially it is worse after exercise but gradually it increases until later it is present at rest and may even awaken the patient from sleep. Pain in the early stages may be due to reactive muscle spasm, to an acute-on-chronic synovitis or to stretching of ligaments or joint capsule by a synovial effusion. It is worth emphasising how quickly the related muscles around an affected joint become involved. Within only a few days quadriceps muscle atrophy may be observed in the vicinity of a knee joint which is the seat of a synovial effusion from whatever cause. In the later stages a dull deep boring pain may supervene and this indicates underlying bone involvement. A further source of pain in a peripheral joint such as hip or knee is a sudden, lancinating, agonising pain which may appear at any time and often interrupts sleep. It is thought that this pain is due to small particles of cartilage or bone which become lodged between the articulating surfaces, producing sudden pain and severe muscle spasm. With our increasing appreciation of the importance of crystal-induced arthritis it is now possible to elicit a history of "gout-like" episodes interrupting the course of osteoarthritis which may be associated with acute joint swelling, redness and severe tenderness.

The stiffness accompanying osteoarthritis is usually less severe and of shorter duration than in inflammatory arthritides such as rheumatoid arthritis.

Loss of function is the complaint which ranks next to pain in patients with osteoarthritis. On occasion this may be the primary problem and may exist alone.

Hip Joint

Certain problems are particular to single joints and must be considered separately. Until the advent of total joint replacement one of the most feared clinical situations was the patient who suffered from severe bilateral hip joint disease. Those patients frequently suffered prolonged agonising pain and the functional disability of bilateral fixed, adducted and flexed hip joints was dreadful. The problems with sexual intercourse and with even simple personal hygiene were formidable. It is in patients such as this that one can best appreciate the importance of reconstructive surgery. Pain from the hip is usually experienced on the inside of the upper thigh and in the groin. Pain above this is more likely to derive from disease in the lumbar spine. If there is any doubt about the source of the pain there is a simple manoeuvre (which does not replace full and proper examination of the joint!) which may be of assistance. With the patient lying supine and the spine and knee flat, place the examining hand on the lower shin. Gently roll the extended leg and if the foot describes a full arc in each direction then it is unlikely that the pain derives from that hip joint. This manoeuvre rolls the femoral head within the acetabulum and usually exposes disease within the cavity of the hip joint. Pain from the hip may also be experienced in the buttocks or over the acetabulum but other possible local causes should first be excluded. Clinical signs of hip joint disease include limitation of movement and apparent shortening of the leg. It is important to examine carefully since true shortening indicates dislocation, collapse of the femoral head or fracture of the neck of femur. A positive Trendelenburg test may be elicited in which the patient walks with an antalgic gait, leaning to the side of the lesion.

Knee Joint

The knee is frequently involved in osteoarthritis and it is interesting that there seem to be racial, geographical and ethnic differences in the frequency of involvement of the hip and knee. Whereas osteoarthritis of the hip is uncommon in people of Chinese extraction, osteoarthritis of the knee is found very commonly in Egyptians. Until properly controlled population studies have been completed such clinical observations rest on an insecure foundation yet may provide useful clues. In the United Kingdom the knee joint is particularly at risk in young persons during sport and repeated damage at this age does seem to predispose to osteoarthritis in later life. It is interesting that meniscectomy, which certainly solves the immediate local problem, seems to be a factor in the later development of osteoarthritis. Osteoarthritis may supervene in those joints which were afflicted by that ill-defined syndrome "chondromalacia patellae" in earlier life and this may explain some cases of isolated arthritis of the patellofemoral compartment. These patients feel pain, particularly on negotiating stairs, and tenderness and grating may be elicited by moving the patella over the femur. There may be a positive patellar test (the patient tightens the quadriceps while the examiner's hand is placed firmly around the lower third of the thigh—N.B. this test must never be performed if the diagnosis is already apparent since it may provoke severe pain!). Some of these patients may have begun life with congenital abnormalities of the patellar tendon and others may have been hypermobile in their earlier years. Approximately 6% of the population are hypermobile and the great majority of these come to no harm. Indeed, this attribute may prove to be a positive asset if the person happens to wish to become a ballet dancer. On the other hand a few do develop premature osteoarthritis and in a minute proportion the characteristic indicates an underlying genetically determined inborn error of matrix metabolism such as

Marfan's syndrome or one of the many variants of the Ehlers-Danlos syndrome (Tables 2.1, 2.2).

More commonly osteoarthritis of the knee affects the tibiofemoral joint. Whether or not obesity plays a part in the genesis of osteoarthritis of the knee may be debatable, but there is no doubt that obesity exacerbates the symptoms of established disease and, more importantly, that weight reduction will result in a reduction in these symptoms. Osteoarthritis of the knee is particularly prevalent in patients with maturity-onset [type 2] diabetes mellitus but the reason for the association may reside more in the accompanying obesity than in the diabetes itself. Whatever the precise reason, weight reduction will benefit the patient from both points of view.

Clinically the affected knee will be painful and swelling may be due both to bony enlargement and to underlying synovial effusion. The surrounding muscles, in particular the vastus medialis which bears the brunt of disuse atrophy in this instance, will be wasted. There may be tenderness clearly located along the articular margin and there may be a flexion, valgus or varus deformity. The most important point to emphasise about flexion deformities in this, as in any peripheral joint, is the importance of prevention rather than treatment of the established deformity. When any peripheral joint is injured or inflamed there is a natural tendency to hold that joint in flexion, which provides immediate pain relief. When the cause of the pain is removed, however, that joint is then in a disadvantageous position from the point of view of subsequent function and this is easily taught to nurses and medical students by asking them to walk about with their knee joint held in only a few degrees of flexion. It becomes obvious that immense abnormal load is then placed upon the opposite hip and knee and the lower lumbar spine. In time this deformity itself will produce disease in these other areas—"long leg arthropathy". This is a lesson of fundamental importance for all involved in the care of patients of all ages afflicted with any form of arthritis and is of particular importance to the nursing and the physiotherapy care. The point is of such importance that it should be emphasised to every patient at the earliest stage in their disease.

A further point of general importance which may be considered at this stage is joint rupture. Any joint which is the seat of a synovial effusion, and even a joint which was previously apparently normal may undergo this complication, and far from being rare this is one of the most common misdiagnoses encountered by the rheumatologist. The clinical presentation is of a patient with a swollen, tender calf who may also have slight swelling of that ankle and a positive Homans' sign. The calf may be swollen, tender, warm to the touch and even red, denoting local inflammation. The diagnosis reached by the medical attendant is either local sepsis or a deep vein thrombosis and inappropriate antibiotic or anticolagulant therapy is instituted to the detriment of the patient. As is often the case, the clue lies in the history. The patient will often state that his knee joint was swollen. He then felt a sudden pain in the back of the knee or calf "as if I had been kicked, doctor". Even in the absence of such a clear-cut history it is nevertheless important to keep in mind the possibility of joint rupture with outpouring of irritant synovial fluid into the soft tissue planes of the calf since this is such a common occurrence. The diagnosis may be confirmed by ultrasound or by arthrography when radio-opaque contrast medium (water-soluble, e.g. metrizamide) injected into the articular cavity may be seen leaking into the calf. If the procedure is performed too long after the event the gap may have sealed, producing a false-negative result. Alternatively ultrasound techniques can demonstrate fluid planes in calf muscle. On occasion deep venous thrombosis and joint rupture may coexist and this may be demonstrated by a combination of arthrography and phlebography.

The management of a joint rupture is to splint the joint in the position of maximum function in the first instance. Often this, together with reassurance and withdrawal of unnecessary medications, is all that is required. Patients who do not respond may benefit from one of the NSAIDs, and lavage and injection of a small dose of a corticosteroid preparation will produce relief in the unusual event of persisting symptoms.

Examination of the knee includes examination of the important surrounding and internal ligaments. The anterior and posterior cruciate ligaments are tested with the hip and knee flexed and the foot stabilised. The collateral ligaments are examined with the knee in 10–15° of flexion to avoid the problem of locking of the fully extended knee. The integrity of the menisci is established by slow and gentle extension of the flexed knee with the foot either fully inverted or everted. It is worth restating at this juncture the importance of precision in the history and clinical examination and of determining the site of maximal tenderness exactly (Fig 1.1). It is also worth re-emphasising that examination of any joint should begin with the functional ability of that joint and that the opposite joint and the joint above and below the affected joint should be examined first. Any person who concludes the examination of the knee without observing the patient walking and climbing stairs deserves the problems which he will undoubtedly encounter although his patients do not.

Ankle and Foot

In the foot the first metatarsophalangeal joint is frequently involved. Hallux valgus is very common, as is the stiff toe of hallux rigidus. A small point but one worth making to the neurologist is the unreliability of the plantar toe reflex in such patients. Even in the presence of definite long tract signs the response may be equivocal or flexor if there is severe disease of this joint. Whether or not it might be possible to prevent osteoarthritis in this joint by the use of sensible footwear in the early years of life is unlikely to be answered until someone divines a way of inducing the female of the species to eschew the habit of following fashion. The only therapeutic initiative of value in established cases is surgical.

The ankle joint and the other joints of the foot are only rarely afflicted by osteoarthritis unless there has previously been injury or disease. Osteochondritis is an example of the latter.

Upper Limb

Osteoarthritis of the upper limb is much less of a problem than in the lower limb. Osteoarthritis of the shoulder is so uncommon that its presence should immediately raise the suspicion of an underlying infection, inflammatory arthritis or metabolic disease. Crystal arthritis and very rarely ochronosis may affect the shoulder in this way. In the elbow osteoarthritis may occur as a complication of a previous malunited fracture, as is also the case in the wrist. In fact involvement or non-involvement of the wrist is a very useful clinical sign. If the wrist joint itself is tender over the joint margin then it is likely that the pathology is an inflammatory synovitis since it is so seldom involved in osteoarthritis alone. The opposite of this is pain in the carpometacar-pophalangeal joint of the thumb, which indicates the presence of osteoarthritis rather than rheumatoid arthritis (which nearly always spares this joint). Although generally more of a nuisance than a serious disability, osteoarthritis of this joint in the thumb can assume catastrophic dimensions in certain patients, in particular professional golfers, dentists and concert pianists. Rarely in such circumstances operative intervention may be required.

Involvement of the carpal and metacarpal joints is conspicuously less common in osteoarthritis compared with rheumatoid arthritis. The second and third metacarpal joints may be involved in primary generalised osteoarthritis, in calcium pyrophosphate arthritis and in the arthritis associated with haemochromatosis. Bony enlargement of the proximal interphalangeal joints is described by the eponym "Bouchard's" nodes whereas the equivalent in the distal joint is known as "Heberden's" nodes. These may present quite acutely, often around the time of the menopause, with all of the associated clinical signs of an inflammatory reaction. In such cases it is often worth excluding an underlying crystal synovitis. Even in these circumstances the long-term prognosis is excellent and the most important part of management is firm reassurance, coupled with the most important part of the physician's art, namely keeping the patient amused whilst Nature cures the disease.

Osteoarthritis is not a diagnosis but a description. Before applying this term the physician should reassure himself that there are no signs of constitutional or systemic involvement, that the haemoglobin concentration and ESR are normal and that any synovial fluid aspirated is non-inflammatory in nature and sterile. The cell count should not be grossly elevated, the fluid should have retained some elements of its viscous properties and a search for crystals of urate or pyrophosphate should have been negative. Radiological examination will reveal loss of joint "space", subchondral sclerosis and cysts (geodes), peaking of the tibial spines in the knee and marginal osteophytosis.

Management

Management of a patient with osteoarthritis is geared to the individual. Certain general principles apply. No patient can be hurt by the general advice to attain and maintain their maximum physical fitness and mobility. Weight gain should be discouraged and weight reduction, where necessary, should be gradual. It is ironic that one of the consequences of injudicious hasty weight reduction should be the precipitation of gouty arthritis.

Secondary prevention is also of importance. Excessive use of an affected joint should be curtailed, but in the present economic climate a difficult balance must often be struck between this on the one hand and loss of an essential job on the other. In the case of the hip joint much relief may be obtained by the use of a walking stick held in the hand on the side opposite to that of the affected joint. The importance of avoiding flexion deformities bears reiteration and it is also worth emphasising that whilst treating the affected joint, prevention of subsequent episodes in that and in other joints is of equal importance. The balance between rest of an actively involved joint and the need for subsequent mobilisation of that joint and for preservation of mobility in all other areas must be carefully struck for the individual patient. When splinting is used it is vital that this be in the optimum position for the individual joint. Many of the accoutrements of physical medicine are at best untested or at worst already proven to be useless. Wax baths, the application of various forms of electrical or thermal energy and counter-irritants applied to the skin are of symptomatic value only.

Selection of Drug Therapy (covered in full in Chaps. 13, 14)

It is important to emphasise that these are symptomatic remedies and that therefore the patient is the only person who is in a position to make the final decision. It is also important to emphasise that no drug will abolish pain safely and that the therapeutic goal is to reduce pain to a level with which the patient can cope. It is also sensible to attempt to limit drug therapy to only one drug at a time, which makes it easier to judge both the efficacy and the significance of adverse reactions. Finally it is important to minimise both the daily dose and the total dose. Whenever possible, patients should avoid drug therapy. Patients often ask whether or not they should continue to take their regular drug therapy even when they are feeling quite comfortable and the answer to this question should now be perfectly obvious. These drugs are prescribed only with the object of relieving symptoms. There is no sense whatsoever in continuing to take the drug in the absence of symptoms. In addition there is increasing evidence of a disquieting nature to suggest that the NSAIDs may produce long-term adverse effects in a wide variety of organs and tissues and on various cellular functions, including renal function and calcium and bone metabolism, providing additional reason for caution. These drugs are being overprescribed at present. It is important that the physician adopts a more discriminating and cautious approach. Such considerations make it even more important to focus attention upon non-drug management.

Non-drug Management

One therapeutic modality which is of considerable value to the patient but which is presently abused is physiotherapy. Many thousands of patients are now attending physiotherapy out-patient departments on a regular basis, deriving no benefit whatsoever yet costing the restricted resources of the health service dearly. In large measure this results from a combination of inadequate assessment of available treatment methods combined with failure to construct a rational and attainable therapeutic goal. The only therapeutic measures of proven long-term value in the field of physiotherapy are rest and exercise. The value of judicious local and general exercise is underrated and finds its most clear-cut application pre- and postoperatively. Hydrotherapy is one very convenient method of maximising the value of exercise whilst protecting the patient from the articular consequences of irregular repetitive impulse loading. We are fortunate in the United Kingdom in having convenient access to public swimming baths for most patients and this should be the first step. Thereafter the role of the physiotherapist should be primarily educative in nature. Each patient should receive instruction in the exercise programme most appropriate to that individual and once the physiotherapist has satisfied herself that the patient understands, then it is the responsibility of the individual to continue this programme on a regular basis. Symptomatic measures such as local heat, however applied, are of value only inasmuch as they facilitate this exercise programme.

The physiotherapist, the occupational therapist, the social worker, the disablement resettlement officer and the appliance officer can all provide essential services in individual cases and the relief afforded by access to a competent and interested chiropodist may be enormous. It is therefore vitally important that the general practitioner and/or the local consultant physician should be thoroughly aware of the potential contribution which these colleagues are in a position to make. It is equally important that he understand the limitations of these disciplines. For example, in the field of functional aids in the kitchen and bathroom the judicious prescription of the appropriate aid for the individal may transform that patient's life and allow the patient to perform tasks for which he or she would otherwise have to rely upon others. On the other hand a vast amount of money is wasted upon aids which patients find to be absolutely useless. Sometimes the aid which the patient finds to be most useful is the aid which he has designed himself.

A similar situation obtains when considering footwear. Patients with all forms of arthritis find great difficulty in finding suitable footwear and the art of making shoes to individual specification is a dying art. Too few of the younger generation are learning the techniques required and the cost of individualised footwear is rising sharply. A great deal of money is presently being wasted in providing footwear for patients who find the product to be unacceptable either in terms of comfort or cosmesis and these expensive shoes simply languish unused in patients' cupboards at home. With the availability of modified plastics it should soon be possible to provide much more suitable cosmetically acceptable shoes at low cost. It has been estimated that as much as 4 million pounds sterling may be saved in this way annually, emphasising the importance of this subject.

Once all of these general principles have been explored and all potentially treatable co-diseases such as anaemia, hypothyroidism and depression have been excluded, one is sometimes left in the position of having a patient who is well controlled in all respects with the exception of a single or a few index joints. Here the possibility of surgical intervention may arise if the joint in question is surgically accessible. This topic is covered in detail in Chap. 19. It is worth emphasising that a close liaison between the physician and the surgeon is absolutely vital, whether this be in the form of a "combined clinic" or in a less formal context. The indications for surgical intervention are unremitting pain and functional impairment, and the morale and motivation of the patient are of paramount importance.

In certain circumstances the patient may present a problem midway between these two extremes. One joint may be troublesome which is either surgically inaccessible or which is not so severely involved as to justify surgery. Here the question of injection may be raised. A recent review which went to great lengths to take into account all of the available evidence concluded that it is not justifiable to inject osteoarthritic joints with corticosteroid. On the other hand there is no doubt that a synovial effusion in, for example, the knee will itself interfere with joint function and will produce atrophy of the related quadriceps muscles. The question must be resolved by the attending physician and requires balanced judgement. A large persistent synovial effusion unresponsive to other methods of management provides an indication for joint aspiration and lavage undertaken with full aseptic precautions. The fluid must be sent for bacteriological and crystallographic examination and a sample should be examined at the time for appearance, viscosity and cell count and typing. Much benefit may accrue from this alone. If anything further is required then the possibility of additional injection of corticosteroid may be considered.

Further Reading

Bland JH, Stulberg SD (1981) Osteoarthritis; pathology and clinical patterns. In: Kelly W, Harris ED Jr, Ruddy S, Sledge CB (eds) Textbook of rheumatology, 1st edn. Saunders, Philadelphia London Toronto, Chap 89

Brandt KD (1981) Glycosaminoglycans. In: Kelly W, Harris ED Jr, Ruddy S, Sledge CB (eds) Textbook of rheumatology, 1st edn. Saunders, Philadelphia London Toronto, Chap 88

Brandt KD (1981) Pathogenesis of osteoarthritis. In: Kelly W, Harris ED Jr, Ruddy S, Sledge CB (eds) Textbook of rheumatology, 1st edn. Saunders, Philadelphia London Toronto, Chap 88

Brooks PM, Potter SR, Buchanan WW (1982) NSAID and osteoarthritis — help or hindrance? J Rheumatol 9: 3–5

Harris ED (1981) Biology of the joint. In: Kelly W, Harris ED Jr, Ruddy S, Sledge CB (eds) Textbook of rheumatology, 1st edn. Saunders, Philadelphia London Toronto, Chap 18

Jiminez SA, Lally EV (1980) Disorders of collagen structure and metabolism. Bull Rheum Dis 3–4: 1016–1022

Kwang AH (1981) Connective tissue; collagen and elastin. In: Kelly W, Harris ED Jr, Ruddy S, Sledge CB (eds) Textbook in rheumatology, 1st edn. Saunders, Philadelphia London Toronto, Chap 16

Lee P, Rooney PJ, Sturrock RD, Kennedy AC, Dick W Carson (1974) The aetiology and pathogenesis of osteoarthritis. Semin Arthritis Rheum 3(3): 189–218

Nuki G (1980) Aetiopathogenesis of osteoarthritis. Pitman Medical, London Tunbridge Wells

Robinson WD (1981) Management of degenerative joint disease. In: Kelly W, Harris ED Jr, Ruddy S, Sledge CB (eds) Textbook in rheumatology, 1st edn. Saunders, Philadelphia London Toronto, Chap 90

Young A, Hughes I, Round JM, Edwards RHT (1982) The effect of knee injury on the number of muscle fibres in the quadriceps femoris. Clin Sci 62: 227–234

3 Pain in the Neck, Low Back Pain and Degenerative Disc Disease

Pain in the Neck

Pain in the neck is common and is the cause of considerable morbidity. This clinical syndrome has various causes:

1. *Infection*: pyogenic, tuberculosis, meningitis
2. *Inflammation*: seronegative spondarthritides, rheumatoid arthritis
3. *Degenerative*: osteoarthritis, degenerative disc disease
4. *Structural*: cervical rib, cervical canal stenosis
5. *Metabolic*: osteopenia, osteomalacia
6. *Trauma*: fracture, non-articular strain, "whiplash injury"
7. *Non-specific pain*: soft tissue rheumatism, postural, "psychogenic"
8. *Referred pain*: retropharyngeal pathology
9. *Neoplastic*: secondary, primary (intra- or extramedullary lesion)

The cervical spine of all mammals, including even the giraffe, has seven vertebrae. Like the lumbar spine, it has a protective and supportive role. The cervical spine, however, is very mobile, allowing movement in six planes. Apart from the central articulations (the secondary cartilaginous joints or symphyses, which are devoid of synovium), there are two diarthrodial joints between each spinal segment. The facet joints are set at an angle of 45° which permits a compromise between movement and stability, and in addition the neurocentral joints at the margins of the disc are synovial lined. The vertebrae protect the spinal cord and the vertebral arteries ascending through the intervertebral foramina.

The skull rests upon the atlas and both rotational and flexion/extension movements occur here. The atlas has no vertebral body but instead the odontoid process of the axis is held between the anterior face of the bone and the transverse ligament. Synovial bursae separate the process from the ligament and this is an area of considerable importance in inflammatory diseases such as rheumatoid arthritis or ankylosing spondylitis.

The term "cervical spondylosis" is used to include the process involved in both disc degeneration and osteoarthritis of the spine, expressing the close relationship between these two diseases. Each alone or together is responsible for a large proportion of episodes of neck pain. The pain is usually described as dull or aching, may be exacerbated by movement (sometimes in a particular direction) and is usually worse in the evenings or at night. Sleep may be impaired and often the patient will complain of pain on awakening. A characteristic feature of cervical spine disease is pain which begins at the occiput then radiates over the vertex and settles in the frontal area. This indicates involvement of the cervical nerve roots. It is obviously important to consider in the differential diagnosis all other causes of headache, the more so when one recognises the insecurity of finding changes on radiological examination of the cervical spine. Many symptomless patients have X-ray changes and the most dangerous trap is to ascribe the clinical symptoms wrongly to osteoarthritis in the presence of much more serious pathology. It is worth stating the obvious: when changes in the cervical spine become radiologically apparent they have already been present for a considerable time and caution should be exercised before ascribing recent symptoms to them. It is also important to remember iatrogenesis. The very drugs prescribed for headache and neck pain themselves may produce these symptoms and all that is required is to remove the offending agent. Indomethacin is the best recognised in this context but most other NSAIDs may also produce this side-effect.

Well-known clues indicating the possibility of disc protrusion, such as exacerbation of symptoms with coughing, sneezing or straining at stool, require little emphasis, but simple useful clinical tests are often neglected. Production or exacerbation of symptoms by positional change such as flexion (which suggests disc protrusion), extension (which suggests facet joint disease) or tilting to one or other side (which suggests osteophytic or disc encroachment) is often omitted, as is a search for local paravertebral muscle spasm. The value of these tests is enhanced considerably when the manoeuvre also produces distinct dysaesthesia along the territory of a particular nerve or root. The dermatome and peripheral nerve distributions are illustrated in Tables 3.1 and 3.2. It is too often stated that the clinical picture may be confused by multiple level involvement and by vascular involvement and this is often true. More often, however, it is an excuse for careless clinical practice. The importance of attempting to localise the lesion is underlined by the all-too-common patient who presents for cervical fusion with the scars of unsuccessful surgical intervention at the wrist and elbow clearly evident. There are better ways to localise the level of involvement than multiple surgical exploration.

A common clinical problem is the patient who presents with pain in the shoulder but whose symptoms owe their genesis to disease in the cervical spine. This is the counterpart of the similar problem of referred pain discussed above in the context of the lower limb. The first clue arises during

Table 3.1. Anatomy of cervical roots

Root	Sensory area	Muscles	Reflex
C5	Radial aspect forearm	Shoulder abductors Elbow flexors	Biceps
C6	Radial side of hand, thumb and index finger	Wrist extensors and pronators	Supinator
C7	Back of forearm, hand and middle finger	Extensors, elbow and fingers	Triceps
C8	Ulnar aspect hand and little finger	Flexors of wrist and fingers	
T1	Ulnar border forearm	Small muscles of hand	

the clinical examination, when the symptoms are exacerbated by rotation or tilting of the head. The second is simply to ask the patient to place his or her hand over the pain. If the hand is placed over the clavicle or above, then the source of the problem is in the neck. If the hand is placed over the deltoid insertion, then it is likely that the pain does indeed stem from the shoulder itself. Confirmation may be obtained by finding clinical clues to the presence of disease in or around the shoulder. A further clinical clue of inestimable value is the presence of distinct and prolonged stiffness in the morning and after inactivity, indicating the presence of one of the inflammatory arthritides.

The first step in the management of a patient with pain in the neck, therefore, is precision in diagnosis and assessment. Thereafter all of the general principles discussed above with reference to peripheral joint disease find equally important application. Reassurance, removal of treatable complications and co-diseases, and non-specific general measures are again more important than the selection of an antirheumatic drug. With particular reference to the neck, advice to alter inappropriate sleeping positions and the correct use of pillows may suffice; the following guidelines are given:

1. Maintain a good posture, with your head, neck and chest in a straight line
2. At night use only one pillow
3. Avoid carrying heavy weights by hand
4. Support arms on a chair rest when sitting
5. Avoid the stooping posture
6. Perform exercises three or four times daily to mobilise the neck and to strengthen the neck and shoulder muscles

The balance between rest and exercise is again important, and the general rule is that the only thing which will relieve acute pain is rest and time. Thereafter as soon as the pain is relieved the patient should be encouraged to commence a graduated, carefully supervised exercise programme directed both generally and locally. Swimming is one of the simplest and best therapeutic modalities. The purpose of the programme is secondary prevention and this must be explained to the patient. It is worth emphasising that activity, involvement and the attainment and maintenance of the patient's maximum physical fitness and mobility are the cornerstones of management. The practice of simply dismissing the patient with an inappropriate and ill-fitting cervical collar is to be deprecated. If a collar is indicated because of persisting pain, it must be properly fitted to achieve the dual role of comfort for the patient and partial immobilisation of the neck. As soon as the acute episode is over, the collar should be discarded, except in a few elderly addicted patients or in those patients who derive benefit and in particular achieve an otherwise impossible night's sleep from this measure. Unnecessary long-term use of collars should be discouraged since it interferes with a mobilisation programme, encourages the patient in invalidism and dependency and predisposes to vertebral osteopenia and loss of muscle tone.

There remains a numerically small but clinically important group of patients who do not respond to these measures. In the presence of unremitting pain or in particular of advancing neurological symptoms and signs, continuous cervical traction may be required. It hardly requires stating that this carries a potential morbidity and extreme caution is required. These patients require admission and the availability of a fully trained and interested nursing staff is essential. In this situation and in that further group of less acute but nevertheless non-responding patients, close consultation with the surgeon is again mandatory. The most unequivocal indication for surgical intervention is the surgical emergency of a central disc prolapse with local pain, neurological signs and sphincter disturbance. In the other group of more chronic patients the indications are less clear and individual judgement is critical. The surgeon likes to see a situation where there is a clear-cut local and focal lesion, and it is in such cases that the best results are obtained from operation. The further the clinical situation departs from this, the worse become the results. The most serious error is in failure of assessment, and here an evaluation of the patient's personality and previous response to adversity and pain must be included.

It is conspicuous that little mention has been made of drug therapy. In fact antirheumatic drugs are often very disappointing in such patients. Pure analgesics may be preferred by the patient but the general principles of selection and prescription apply (p. 16, Chaps. 4, 13). Every attempt should be made to raise the pain threshhold and to minimise the need for drug therapy. The patient should be encouraged to select a single preparation on the basis of patient preference and both daily and total dosage should again be kept to a minimum.

Low Back Pain

Back pain constitutes one of the major reasons for medical consultation, for disability and for time lost from work in the United Kingdom. The experience of low back pain is almost universal, so one of the earliest considerations must be the threshold effect or why that particular patient presented to the doctor at a particular time. The possible causes of back pain are:

1. *Congenital*: deformity, spondylolisthesis, spina bifida
2. *Inflammatory*: infection, e.g. staphylococci, tuberculosis, brucellosis; inflammatory, e.g. seronegative spondarthritides, rheumatoid arthritis; Scheuermann's disease
3. *Mechanical/structural*: spinal canal stenosis, fracture/trauma etc.
4. *Degenerative*: prolapsed disc, osteoarthritis, ankylosing hyperostosis
5. *Metabolic*: osteopenia, osteomalacia, Paget's disease
6. *Neoplastic*: primary, metastatic (bronchus, breast, kidney, thyroid, ovary), haematological (reticulosis, myeloma)
7. *Referred*: renal, pancreatic, gastrointestinal, ovarian, uterine, vascular

Of the above categories, by far the most important are mechanical and structural, including osteoarthritis and degenerative disc disease, metabolic bone disease and inflammatory arthritides such as ankylosing spondylitis. The general principles referred to above serve to distinguish one from the other in the vast majority of cases and again the clinical history and examination are of paramount importance.

The lumbar spine serves three functions: (a) support, (b) protection of the spinal canal, cauda equina and emerging nerve roots and (c) fulcrum for the great muscles of the trunk and lower limbs. There are five lumbar vertebrae positioned in a lordotic curve and connected by the secondary cartilaginous symphyses and by the diarthrodial joints, the facet joints. These latter joints are set at a more acute angle than in the cervical spine, reflecting the greater importance of stability over mobility at this level. The facet joints protect the disc from torsional and rotational strains and the spinal segments are bound together very firmly by immensely powerful anterior and posterior spinal ligaments, the ligamentum flavum and the paravertebral muscles.

The intervertebral disc consists of the incompressible proteoglycan-rich nucleus pulposus and the concentrically arranged collagenous annulus fibrosus. The nucleus has the properties required to distribute forces equally in all directions. The collagen fibres in the annulus are arranged diagonally as well as concentrically, allowing this structure to withstand enormous pressures. Since these structures are avascular, nutrition occurs by diffusion from peripheral blood vessels.

In the standing position the weight of the body is balanced by the supportive function of the sum of these spinal "mobile segments", with each disc acting as a fulcrum. Any increased load must be met by these structures to the point of failure. At that point disc material may be extruded vertically through the vertebral plate to form a Schmorl's node or horizontally. It is an oversimplification to use the term "a slipped disc" since this is not in fact what happens. Rather there is protrusion of peripheral disc material which again is usually itself abnormal prior to this event. Measurement of intradiscal pressure has been accomplished both in normal subjects and in various disease states. At the level of L-3 pressure is least when the subject is lying supine; it increases on sitting (especially when "sagging"), standing and bending forwards and changes dramatically when the subject is attempting to lift even a light object with the knees straight. It is on the basis of data such as these that our present advice on care of the back rests.

Instructions to patients with back pain:
A straight spine puts less pressure on the individual discs; therefore always keep the spine straight, especially standing, sitting and lying. It may help to rest one foot on a rail when standing.

Do not
Lift weight above head
Stoop
Move furniture or similar weights
Push windows up
Put on weight
Get over-tired
Stand or sit in one position for a long time.

Do
Sleep on a firm mattress with one pillow
Support the back whilst driving a car
Lift objects from the ground by bending the knees and holding object close to body
Avoid activities that would strain the back
Adapt work to keep back straight and pain free

Prevention of back pain:
1. Education of school children in principles of back care
2. Screening of at risk groups prior to employment
3. Changes in industry to avoid back damage, with special powers given to work safety committees to enforce them
4. Statutory weights which people may lift, as recommended by The International Labour Organisation
5. Adaption to working conditions to prevent stooping
6. Attention to general fitness

Booklets provided by organisations such as the Arthritis and Rheumatism Council are invaluable aids to patient communication in this as in many other areas, particularly when one bears in mind how little information a patient takes away from even the most skilled medical communicator. In addition information such as this should prove to be helpful in future designs of car and work seats which are today woefully inadequate.

Although the mechanism of pain production has not yet been fully defined, there are no nerve fibres in the disc. Pain must therefore originate from surrounding ligaments and other soft tissues or from the bony vertebral bodies. Acute low back pain is an alarming experience for the patient. There may be a clear relationship to trauma but often the apparent precipitant appears trivial in nature, strengthening the argument that the disc may previously have been abnormal. The pain is usually described as "knife-like" and may radiate up the spine or down into the buttocks. There is often pronounced paravertebral muscle spasm but the presence of severe or prolonged stiffness should alert the clinician to the possibility of one of the inflammatory spondarthritides. Percussion of each vertebral body and space individually with a tendon hammer may assist in localisation. The clinical signs and symptoms of lumbar disc disease are:

1. Pain in the back at rest, with or without radiation into the thigh or leg
2. Pain increased by movement
3. Reflex scoliosis
4. Paravertebral muscle spasm
5. Straightening out of normal lumbar lordosis
6. Localised tenderness (elicited by palpation or percussion)
7. Restricted movement (often in only one or two planes)
8. Dysaesthesia along the root distribution

In the great majority of cases the problem is confined to the musculoskeletal system but it is important to search for the clinical features which indicate neurological involvement, whether this be radicular, central or peripheral. The dermatome and peripheral nerve distributions are recorded in Table 3.2. Again it is important to attempt to achieve precision in every instance, but as in the cervical spine the problem is often confounded by involvement at multiple levels. The details of clinical examination are covered elsewhere, but it is worth recording one error which is frequently encountered with reference to testing of muscle power in the lower limb. The power of the lower limb musculature in young or middle-aged male or female patients exceeds by far the power of the upper limb musculature of the examiner. There is no point in participating in an undignified trial of strength of the physician's upper limbs against the patient's more powerful lower limbs on the bed. If the patient can stand on tiptoe ten times taking his or her full weight on one foot at a time, and if he or she can walk across the room on their heels then it is likely that the neuromuscular function of the lower limbs is intact. Examination of the power of the extensor hallucis longus muscle on both sides will provide useful clinical information in those patients with evidence of involvement.

A question posed frequently is whether or not a rectal examination should

Table 3.2. Localisation of disc protrusion

Root	Sensory Area	Muscles involved	Reflex
L2	Upper thigh	Hip flexors and adductors	None
L3	Anterior surface lower thigh and anterior/medial surface of knee	Hip adductors, knee extensors	Knee possible
L4	Anterior/medial surface leg	Knee extensors, dorsiflexion and inversion foot	Knee
L5	Anterior/lateral surface leg, dorsum foot and great toe	Hip extensors and abductors, knee flexors, dorsiflexion foot and great toe	None
S1	Lateral border and sole foot	Knee flexors, plantar flexion and eversion of foot	Ankle

be performed. In the same manner as for estimation of blood pressure on a routine basis, so the argument may be made that a rectal examination is part of the clinical examination in any adult. However, in the presence of intact lower limb motor and sensory function, including unimpaired sensation in the saddle area, it is difficult to provide any further arguments for rectal examination in the case of an individual suffering from uncomplicated backache.

Management of back pain embodies all of the principles discussed above, both in the context of peripheral arthritis and in the section on pain in the neck. Again, the only measures which are effective in the acute situation are rest in the position of maximum comfort (or least discomfort) and time. Weight control and the attainment and maintenance of the patient's maximum physical fitness and mobility are of central importance. In the context of low back pain the role of the abdominal musculature deserves emphasis since it is this which plays the major part in opposing a rise in intradiscal pressure. The relief afforded by the provision of a lumbar corset is due to this relationship. Wherever possible, it is better for the patient to achieve the desired result by strengthening the abdominal muscle tone actively rather than by the passive effect of a lumbar support. Patients with low back pain often present in their youth or early adult years. At this stage it is worth investing considerable time and effort in education on how to live with a suspect back. This may minimise problems which are likely to occur in later years. In the elderly often palliation is all that can be achieved, but even in this group an attempt at secondary prevention is worthwhile. The increased interest in post-retiral swimming clubs is heartening and should be encouraged. The principles regarding selection and prescription of appropriate drug therapy are identical to those discussed above.

Further Reading

Bland JH, Nakano KK (1981) Neck pain. In: Kelly W, Harris ED Jr, Ruddy S, Sledge CB (eds) Textbook of rheumatology, 1st edn. Saunders, Philadelphia London Toronto, Chap 28

Cyriax J (1978) Textbook of orthopaedic medicine; diagnosis of soft tissue lesions (vol 1). Bailliere Tindall, London

Golub BS, Rovit RL, Mankin HJ (1971) Cervical and lumbar disc disease; a review. Bull Rheum Dis 21: 635–642

Grabias SL, Mankin HJ (1980) Pain in the lower back. Bull Rheum Dis 30: 1040–1045

Hall H (1981) The back doctor. Victor Golanz, London

Jayson MIV (1980) The lumbar spine and back pain. Lippincott, Philadelphia

Lipson SJ (1981) Low back pain. In: Kelly W, Harris ED Jr, Ruddy S, Sledge CB (eds) Textbook of rheumatology, 1st edn. Saunders, Philadelphia London Toronto, Chap 30

Macnab I (1977) Backache. Williams and Williams, Baltimore

Resnick D (1978) Disorders of the axial skeleton which are lesser known, poorly recognised or misunderstood. Bull Rheum Dis 28: 932–939

4 Local Syndromes

Introduction

The physician and especially the medical student tend to view rheumatology from the standpoint of interesting immunological or metabolic disease processes. Thus disproportionate attention is paid to diseases like alkaptonuria or systemic lupus erythematosus. It is certainly of the first importance to be in a position to manage patients with rare diseases competently, and it is incumbent on those who are not regularly exposed to such clinical situations to take the appropriate consultative steps. It is sad that so many patients presenting with rare diseases are often badly advised and treated. On the other hand the common day-to-day problems which arise in rheumatological practice do not fit into this category and it is for this reason that we have devoted so much of this text to the far more common diseases and syndromes.

Some of the most common clinical presentations in rheumatology may be encompassed by the term "local syndromes". The most frequently seen of these is the patient who presents with pain in the region of the shoulder.

Shoulder Syndromes

Painful lesions that occur around the shoulder are:

1. *Musculoskeletal*
   a) Rotator cuff lesions
   b) Calcific tendinitis
   c) Bicipital tendinitis
   d) "Capsulitis"
   e) "Frozen shoulder"

2. *Arthritis*
   a) Inflammatory synovitis
   b) Osteoarthritis (rare—usually secondary)
3. *Trauma*
4. *Referred pain*
   a) Cervical spine
   b) Chest (heart, lungs and pleura)
   c) Gall bladder (right side)
   d) Peritoneum
5. *Shoulder/hand syndrome*

In order to appreciate the significance of symptoms and signs in the shoulder region it is important to understand the anatomy. The shoulder girdle is formed by the scapula and clavicle, which articulate at the acromioclavicular joint. The shoulder girdle itself is attached to the trunk at the sternoclavicular joint. Both of these joints are easily accessible to clinical examination so there is no excuse for omitting this part of the clinical examination. The glenohumeral joint is a "ball and socket" joint, the head of the humerus forming the ball which articulates with the shallow glenoid socket. Stability is compromised in the interests of mobility, which explains the propensity of this joint to dislocate. Stability is subserved by the surrounding ligaments, tendons and muscles. Four muscles are of particular importance, namely, the supraspinatus, infraspinatus, subscapularis and teres minor. Together these form the "rotator cuff".

Closely associated with the shoulder joint is the subacromial bursa, which separates the supraspinatus tendon from the coraco-acromial arch. Although usually a closed space in the normal, communication with the glenohumeral joint cavity may occur in some patients with inflammatory joint disease. The long head of biceps has a tendon sheath which communicates with the glenohumeral cavity. The nerve supply of the shoulder is from branches of the suprascapular, axillary and lateral pectoral nerves and in accordance with neurological principle, these nerves also serve the areas of skin overlying the joint. In particular, the axillary nerve serves the upper lateral aspect of the arm over the insertion of the deltoid muscle, which is a common source of referred pain.

Lesions in and around the shoulder are common causes of consultation both with the general practitioner and with the hospital consultant. The most common reason for consultation is a combination of pain and functional limitation although either may present in isolation. The first step is to ensure that the presenting complaint does indeed have its origin in the region of the shoulder and is not referred pain from the viscera or from the neck. Although this is frequently stressed, in day-to-day clinical practice a combination of positive and negative clinical symptoms and signs usually makes distinction easy. Referred pain is associated with clinical clues to indicate the site or organ initiating the pain together with evidence that the shoulder itself is functioning normally. The distinction between pain deriving from disease in the cervical spine and a shoulder is drawn in Chap. 3.

It is often much more difficult to formulate a precise description in patients who have a painful lesion within the shoulder region itself. Again, the general rule that intra-articular lesions produce painful limitation of movement in *all* directions and planes of movement may be of assistance. Further, expression of a lesion in only one movement or in a restricted combination of movements indicates a lesion of a muscle, tendon, ligament or enthesis. Unfortunately in a considerable proportion of patients the clinical signs and symptoms do not accord with either of these relatively simple situations. The truth is that the pathogenesis and evolution of such syndromes have not been documented and we are woefully ignorant about their aetiology and optimum management. This ignorance is expressed in the words which are used to describe these patients' problems, such as "adhesive capsulitis", "pericapsulitis" and "frozen shoulder". This is an area which would benefit from well-conducted long-term descriptive studies.

The most common lesion affecting the shoulder region is one involving the muscles and tendons of the rotator cuff. This may follow an isolated traumatic episode such as a fall on the outstretched hand or may be a consequence of repeated episodes of microtrauma in industry or in housework. An attempt should be made to define the precise muscle or tendon involved by a sequence of *passive* movements. Involvement of the supraspinatus will cause pain on abduction which may be present only within certain angles of movement, the "painful arc". Pain on external rotation alone indicates involvement of infraspinatus and on internal rotation alone focusses attention on subscapularis. Pain on full passive extension alone suggests involvement of biceps. The initial lesion is usually a tear at the enthesis, the site of insertion of muscle through tendon or ligament into bone. In the case of these muscles around the shoulder the site of insertion often includes the joint capsule. This may in part explain the frequency with which the capsule of this joint is involved and the frequency of occurrence of syndromes with mixed clinical signs. Pain may begin in a predictable localised fashion but may then radiate widely into the arm, making precise diagnosis difficult.

In contrast to the extra-articular lesions which produce pain in particular directions, patients with intra-articular lesions have limitation of movement in all directions and both active and passive movements are affected. As a general principle of joint examination, active and active assisted movements should always be tested before passive movement of a joint is conducted. There is likely to be tenderness along the articular margin and pain deriving from the shoulder joint itself is often experienced at the insertion of the deltoid muscle. The movements which tend to be affected first are lateral rotation and abduction of the glenohumeral joint but thereafter other movements are lost quickly and the picture is described by the evocative term "frozen shoulder". Almost any disease or lesion which tends to immobilise the shoulder may be responsible for the development of this clinical picture, and the vulnerability of the shoulder is probably a consequence of the anatomical compromise between mobility and stability.

Investigation of a shoulder lesion should include an X-ray since this may be of some value. Apart from the occasional fracture or secondary deposit which may be shown, rotator cuff lesions may be marked by roughening of the greater tuberosity and inflammatory synovitis by loss of joint "space"; juxta-articular erosions and local osteopenia and calcific bursitis may also be demonstrated. Calcific bursitis is of considerable interest at present and may be an example of crystal deposition disease. There may be episodes of acute inflammation with severe pain and redness of the overlying skin. The crystal involved is possibly calcium pyrophosphate and/or calcium apatite. The calcification initially may be confined to the tendon but may later spread to involve the closely related bursa; in certain circumstances rupture into the cavity of the glenohumeral joint may occur. Crystal-induced arthritis of the shoulder may be conspicuously destructive.

Whatever the origin of lesion and disease around the shoulder, one of the most important steps in management from the outset (and even earlier if the patient at risk can be identified) is mobilisation. Once immobilised it is likely that whatever the original insult there will be progression to the fully developed picture of a frozen shoulder and the natural history of this is one of a prolonged period of incapacity. Often the patient will be immobilised for a period of 1–2 years despite all attempts at intervention and it is small comfort to such a patient to reassure him or her that the long-term prognosis is very good indeed. It is true that most patients do recover remarkably well after this sort of a delay and that subsequently the function in the affected shoulder is very good indeed. However, a period of 1–2 years of severe incapacity is a very major consideration and every attempt must be made at prevention. It is worth emphasising that patients who have developed frozen shoulder on one side are at greater risk than their fellows of developing it on the other side and are also more liable to develop a wide array of other local syndromes such as nerve entrapment and both low back and cervical spine pain. Thus the presentation of any one of these should alert the clinician to the subsequent development of others of this group and should focus attention on the need to embark upon measures to protect the patient. These are in general perfectly simple and include the need for the patient to avoid excess weight gain and to reduce weight where appropriate, to perform exercises several times daily, putting every joint through a full range of movement, and to attain and maintain maximum physical fitness and mobility. Much can be achieved if the patient swims regularly, if possible two or three times a week.

With particular reference to the presenting painful shoulder joint, the time of first consultation is of paramount importance. If the lesion is caught at the earliest possible moment then a programme of immediate mobilisation of that and of other joints may prevent progression to the fully developed picture. Here swimming or simply movement in warm water can be invaluable.

At this very early stage if there is not an immediate response to early exercise then injection of the appropriate local area, be it intra-articular or extra-articular, may be indicated; however, it must be emphasised that the injection is merely an adjunct to mobilisation and the shoulder should be moved immediately after the injection and repeatedly thereafter. Patients should be encouraged to achieve this by their own active movements, if necessary assisted by the physician. It is unwise to proceed to passive mobilisation at this stage.

The injection into soft tissue should contain initially only the minimum volume of local anaesthetic and no attempt should be made to inject against strong resistance. If the primary problem is intra-articular then the joint cavity should be entered using a wide-bore needle under the same aseptic precautions as are appropriate to the knee or to any other joint. Successive lavage and aspiration of sterile saline should be attempted in the first instance. Very often exercises, swimming and joint aspiration and lavage are sufficient and the problem may be overcome at an early stage.

In those patients who present late or who do not respond to this simple regimen, injection of corticosteroid may be required. One, or at the most two, injections of local corticosteroid will produce sufficient pain relief to allow mobilisation in many of these remaining patients. Again it must be emphasised that corticosteroid should be used only after all simpler and safer methods have been tried first, that corticosteroid should never be introduced into a tendon or ligament and that even corticosteroid represents only an adjunct to the primary management which is mobilisation. One situation where aspiration and local corticosteroid injection may produce particular symptomatic relief is in calcific bursitis, but again the contribution of the aspiration alone may be greater than the specific effect of the corticosteroid.

Other Local Syndromes

Pain due to non-articular disease or trauma is considerably more common than arthritis and indeed is a universal experience. Words like "fibrositis" or "soft tissue rheumatism" are used by patients to describe these situations.

Two considerations are of importance at the outset in considering these local syndromes. In the first place patients who develop one of them are at a higher risk than their fellows of developing others. Very often they occur in previously fit individuals who have become desk-bound, obese and unfit and who attempt to achieve their erstwhile standards without proper preparation. The implications for management are obvious. Secondly these are examples of "time-locked" diseases. Thus, in the great majority of instances there will be a natural tendency for them to improve of their own volition. Yet again the primary management of patients in this category is to reassure them that there is no sinister underlying disease, to impress upon them that their symptoms may be looked upon as warnings that they should improve their overall physical fitness and to protect them from injudicious and expensive exploitation.

Many local syndromes are examples of traumatic enthesopathies. Indeed the most common cause of disorder or disease of the enthesis is traumatic, this being followed by the seronegative spondarthritides in frequency of occurrence.

Tendons are avascular and once damaged take considerably longer to heal than bone or muscle. Thus a sportsman is far more concerned if he damages a tendon or ligament than if he breaks a bone. Once damaged, a tendon or ligament heals by fibrosis and it is not uncommon for secondary calcification to occur, this often being visible on X-ray. Two common sites where this may occur around the elbow are "golfer's elbow" on the medial side at the common flexor origin and "tennis elbow" on the lateral side at the common extensor origin (Table 4.1). Thus in the former there will be highly localised tenderness near the medial humeral epicondyle while in the latter the tenderness will be isolated to the lateral humeral epicondyle. The appropriate local muscle groups will demonstrate pain and weakness when tested and local corticosteroid injection may produce symptomatic relief. It is a fair rule in this field that the longer it has taken to develop a lesion the longer it will take the lesion to remit. Most cases respond to rest of the involved muscle group and exercise of all other muscle groups. If this is to be effective, complete local rest should be enforced in the affected area. In those patients who do not respond to rest it is worth trying first of all a local injection of local anaesthetic alone, but this must be most accurately localised. In the few who do not respond to this, it is permissible to prescribe a local injection of corticosteroid on one or at the very most two occasions and sometimes the effect is gratifying. Once again it is important to emphasise that the injection must be accurately placed, and that corticosteroid should never be introduced into tendon, ligament or skin. One tragic side-effect of local corticosteroid injection is dehiscence of tendon or skin with accompanying functional disability in the case of the former and superficial unsightly scarring in the latter. This can be particularly distressing if the patient is an attractive young female. The simplest precaution is to ensure that the needle point is accurately located and never to inject against firm resistance.

Table 4.1. Localised painful syndromes around the elbow

Location	Disorder
Lateral epicondyle	Tennis elbow
Articular margin	Synovitis of the elbow joint
Olecranon	Bursitis
Ulnar Groove	Neuropathy (e.g. entrapment)
Medial epicondyle	Golfer's elbow

Very rarely patients fail to respond even to these measures and then surgical consultation may be considered. However, even surgical intervention may be disappointing and should not be entertained lightly.

Carpal Tunnel Syndrome

One common local syndrome in the upper limb is carpal tunnel syndrome. This is associated with a distinctive clinical picture with pain and dysaesthesia radiating into the hand and up the arm. These symptoms are characteristically worse at night. The patient, who is often a middle-aged, menopausal female, finds that she can only obtain relief at night by holding her arm out of the bed. In the classical case there is sensory loss in the territory of the median nerve alone, and the power of opponens pollicis and abductor pollicis is reduced. The other intrinsic small muscles of the hand are spared since they are supplied by the ulnar nerve. Tinel's sign is positive, the patient complaining of characteristic dysaesthesia on forced dorsiflexion of the wrist or on percussion over the carpal tunnel with the wrist in a dorsiflexed position. The diagnosis may be confirmed by demonstration of delay in nerve conduction time and latency but there may be a discrepancy between the results of this test and clinical signs and symptoms. Some patients with the most abnormal result have few or even no symptoms whereas other individuals with the full-blown syndrome have normal results. This redoubles the importance of accurate and complete clinical examination and assessment, and it is on the results of this that therapeutic decisions are taken. Where the laboratory results are in accord with these results, confidence is enhanced. It is wise to observe the patient for a short time and to repeat the clinical and nerve conduction studies in doubtful cases.

The conditions which may be associated with the carpal tunnel syndrome are:

Rheumatoid arthritis
Hypothyroidism
Pregnancy
Menstruation
Acromegaly
Amyloidosis
Juvenile chronic polyarthritis
Seronegative spondarthritides
Osteoarthritis (usually coincidental)

It is worth emphasising that in the great majority of instances there is no associated or precipitating disease. The condition which is most frequently missed and which is worth excluding in any doubtful situation is hypothyroidism, in particular since it is so eminently treatable. One of the most common clinical settings is the occurrence of carpal tunnel syndrome in the context of marked recent weight gain and the implications for management are obvious.

Management of the carpal tunnel syndrome is usually perfectly straightforward. In the first instance all precipitating and treatable co-diseases such as thyroid dysfunction or metabolic obesity should be eliminated. The general principles of management of any person with rheumatological disease noted above apply. Thereafter it is worth first trying the effect of one or at the most two injections of local corticosteroid. In the event of failure of reponse to these simple methods, surgical assistance should be sought. Again the patient should be warned that one episode may be the harbinger of another or of one of the related local syndromes, and predisposing factors (in particular metabolic obesity) must be eliminated. The trap of failing to recognise that one or especially two episodes of carpal tunnel syndrome may represent the initial manifestation of an inflammatory polyarthritis such as rheumatoid arthritis must never be forgotten. Clues to this situation are afforded by early morning stiffness, lassitude and exhaustion, and failure to make a fist with ease and to straighten the fingers promptly thereafter. It is worth examining the feet and in particular the metatarsophalangeal joints since these may be involved early.

The median nerve may be trapped at the elbow and the ulnar nerve may be involved either at the wrist or at the elbow. In the latter instance there will be additional involvement of the flexor carpi ulnaris. Neurological entrapment syndromes at the thoracic and pelvic outlets are common and most of these clinical presentations are perfectly straightforward, the only major difficulty being to think of them.

Local Syndromes in the Lower Limb

Other local syndromes may occur in the lower limbs and in particular the knee and ankle are frequently involved in sports injuries. These are common and are the cause of a considerable amount of morbidity. As a reflection of their previous neglect a whole new discipline and society devoted to sports medicine has arisen. It is doubtful if there can be any justification in segregating any particular group from the population and providing these with any form of special treatment. Rather, the growth of this movement should serve as a stimulus to the physician to rectify his previous inadequacy in this field. It can hardly be of other than social significance that a young woman should have sustained her injury or repeated injury whilst engaged in sport as opposed to working in the home and both circumstances deserve the optimum management.

The principles of this subject are no different from the principles of rheumatology in any other arena. The first step in management is a thorough history and detailed general medical and locomotor examination. A clear appreciation of the local anatomy is a prerequisite. The general principles of rest to the painful area and the attainment and maintenance of maximal physical fitness and mobility in all other areas are no different in the case of a ligamentous injury around the knee from any other subject discussed above. Similarly, the avoidance, wherever possible, of meddlesome interference should be stressed. The abuse of local corticosteroid and anaesthetic injection in competitive sportsmen and women is to be deprecated, as is the gross overprescription of phenylbutazone. It should be remembered that the side-effect of agranulocytosis produced by this drug may occur in young persons after brief exposure. There is now no justification whatsoever for the continued use of phenylbutazone in this situation. One of the plethora of NSAIDs presently available will serve the purpose equally well at far less risk. It is likely that a young sportsman with a sports injury would be much better and more safely served by an informed and interested general practitioner than by many of today's aggressive intervention techniques.

A legacy of enthesopathies around the knee joint is the Pellegrini-Stieda syndrome, with radiological evidence of calcification at ligamentous insertion sites. Examination of the knee joint and of the ligaments in and around the knee is discussed above (p. 14) A similar legacy of enthesopathy, whether produced by trauma or by one of the seronegative spondarthritides, may be seen around the ankle. The only movements possible at the ankle joint itself are flexion and extension. Painful lesions in and around the ankle are summarised in Table 4.2. Again, it is important to examine carefully to elicit the site of maximal tenderness, which frequently gives the clue to the diagnosis. If pain is produced not by flexion or extension but by rotation of the foot then it is likely that the source of the problem is in the midtarsal joints. If there is tenderness localised to the plantar aponeurosis and its insertions then the diagnosis is plantar fasciitis. Often the underlying flexor tendons and their sheaths are involved. As in the palm of the hand, it is important to locate the pathological condition precisely. In the palm of the hand there may be inflammation of the soft tissues under the skin alone, as in Dupuytren's disease. This disease may have its counterpart in involvement of the plantar fascia of the foot. There may be an association between these sites of involvement by fibrosis and fibrosing diseases in other parts of the body and it is worth bearing this in mind although multiple involvement is in fact very rare. Finally, there may be involvement both of the tendon sheaths and of the subcutaneous tissue, which may mark the presence of a disease like scleroderma.

Table 4.2. Painful syndromes round the ankle

Location	Disorder
Over the inferior border of the calcaneum	Plantar fasciitis
Over the posterior border of the calcaneum	Achilles tendinitis
Inferior to the lateral malleolus	Tibial sheath tendinitis
Pain on distraction of a ligament	Ligament sprain
Pain on flexion/extension	Intra-articular synovitis
Pain/tenderness localised over bone	? fracture

The management of the most common of these disorders, namely plantar fasciitis, is along the lines of the principles discussed above in the context of lesions involving the ligaments, muscles and tendons of the rotator cuff. Management is again based upon general principles, beginning first with avoidance of precipitating factors, local rest and the prosecution of general physical fitness. Avoidance of weight gain and controlled weight loss are of particular importance in lesions involving weight-bearing areas. Thereafter accurate local installation of anaesthetic or corticosteroid will serve to control the majority of patients who have failed to respond to simple measures. It must be emphasised that injection of the Achilles tendon is contraindicated in view of the high risk of rupture.

These local syndromes are very common and in many instances they are rewarding to treat. A minimum of knowledge of the relevant anatomy is required. Only after general principles have been explored fully should drug therapy be considered.

Further Reading

Bland JH, Merrit JA, Boushey DR (1977) The painful shoulder. Semin Arthritis Rheum 7(1): 21–47

Corrigan B, Maitland GD (1983) Practical orthopaedic medicine, 1st edn. Butterworths, London

Critchley EMR, Vakil D, Hayward HW, Owen VMH (1976) Dupuytren's disease in epilepsy. J Neurol Neurosurg Psychiatry 39: 498–503

Dixon AStJ (1979) Soft tissue rheumatism. Saunders, Philadelphia London Toronto (Clin Rheum Dis, Vol 5/3)

Gerster J-C, Lagier R, Boivin G (1982) Olecranon bursitis related to C.P.P.D.; clinical and pathologic study. Arthritis Rheum 25: 989–996

Hazlemann BL, Laurin CA, Tremblay GR (1981) The injured joint with a normal X-ray. In: Kelly W, Harris ED Jr, Ruddy S, Sledge CB (eds) Textbook of rheumatology, 1st edn. Saunders, Philadelphia London Toronto, Chap 111

Kay NRM (1981) The clinical diagnosis and management of frozen shoulders. Practitioner 225: 164–172

Nakano KK (1981) Entrapment neuropathies. In: Kelly W, Harris ED Jr, Ruddy S, Sledge CB (eds) Textbook of rheumatology, 1st edn. Saunders, Philadelphia London Toronto, Chap 110

Smythe HA (1981) Fibrositis and other diffuse musculoskeletal disorders. In: Kelly W, Harris ED Jr, Ruddy S, Sledge CB (eds) Textbook of rheumatology, 1st edn. Saunders, Philadelphia London Toronto, Chap 32

Weiss J (1981) The painful shoulder. In: Kelly W, Harris ED Jr, Ruddy S, Sledge CB (eds) Textbook in rheumatology, 1st edn. Saunders, Philadelphia London Toronto, Chap 29

Wood B (1981) The painful foot. In: Kelly W, Harris ED Jr, Ruddy S, Sledge CB (eds) Textbook in rheumatology, 1st edn. Saunders, Philadelphia London Toronto, Chap 31

5 Metabolic Bone Disease

Introduction

Since so many patients with bone disease present to the rheumatologist we have devoted a chapter to this subject. No attempt has been made to cover the disorders of calcium homeostasis, which are properly and fully covered in textbooks of endocrinology and metabolic and renal medicine and in the large rheumatology texts. The diseases of bone which are of most importance to the rheumatologist are osteomalacia, osteopenia (osteoporosis) and Paget's disease, and it is upon these that we have concentrated. In keeping with the rest of this text, we have focussed upon therapeutic implications.

Osteomalacia

Osteomalacia is usually the result of inadequate intake or inadequate absorption of vitamin D and calcium but more and more patients are developing this disease as a result of iatrogenesis. The drugs which may be responsible include diphosphonates, hydantoins and barbiturates. Renal disease results in impairment of the second hydroxylation of vitamin D (the first having taken place in the hepatocyte), with failure to generate the biologically active 1,25-dihydroxycholecalciferol. In children the result is rickets but in the adult a disproportionate reduction in the ratio of bone salt to bone matrix follows. As we learn more about bone histopathlogy it is becoming increasingly obvious that osteomalacia frequently coexists with osteopenia. The usual presentation is with bone pain or fracture but it is important to be alert for the patient who presents with a proximal myopathy and the classical "waddling" gait.

Treatment is to define and treat the underlying disease and thereafter to institute replacement therapy. Cholecalciferol is given as its analogue ergocalciferol and 1,25-dihydroxycholecalciferol as its analogue 1-α-hydroxy-cholecalciferol.

Dietary deficiency is corrected and supplemental vitamin D tablets may be prescribed together with calcium. A dose of 25–125 μg calciferol is needed daily, and some patients require more than this. Vitamin D deficiency states require doses of 7.5–15 mg parenterally monthly or 1α-hydroxycholecal-ciferol orally in a dose of 5 μg daily. In the latter case it must be remembered to reduce the dose as healing progresses. Osteomalacia due to renal disease should be treated with 1α-hydroxycholecalciferol starting with a dose of 1.5 μg daily orally and reducing to a maintenance dose of about 0.5 μg per day.

Monitoring of treatment is by serum calcium and alkaline phosphatase levels and in the final analysis by radiology.

Osteopenia

The proportionate loss of bone matrix and mineral is a feature of the ageing skeleton although it may be influenced in large measure by events which have occurred in early adult life or even in childhood. The dimensions of the problem in this country are enormous and are displayed in the numbers of patients attending the casualty departments with fractures and the orthopaedic and rheumatology departments with back pain. Maximal skeletal bone mass is attained in early adult life and thereafter there is a slow decline in everybody (Fig. 5.1). When a patient develops symptoms and signs attributable to osteopenia then they have crossed the threshold shown in the figure and this is variable from individual to individual. The rate of decline is greater in the

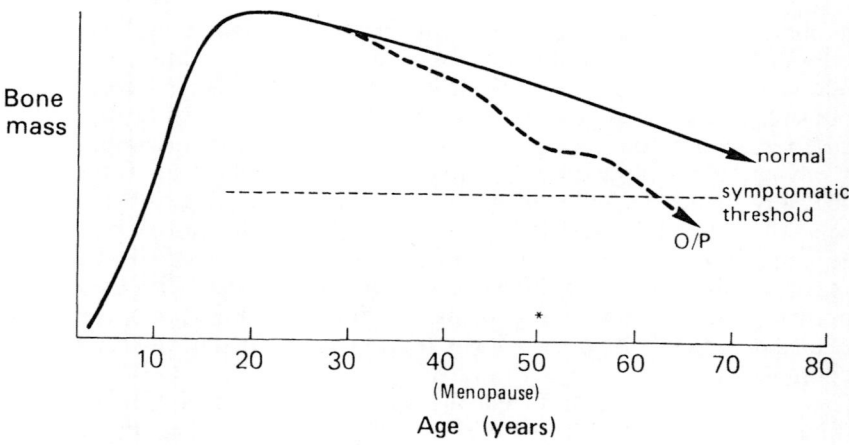

Fig. 5.1. Total bone mass throughout life

female and accelerates for a time during the menopause, accounting for the phrase "postmenopausal" osteopenia. Systemic disease such as rheumatoid arthritis contributes to an increase in the rate of bone loss and corticosteroid therapy exerts an additional and separable effect.

The process is not a simple loss, but rather the dynamic physiological balance between deposition and removal is tilted to the negative side. Indeed, deposition in the most severely affected patients may be increased. The loss of bone is not uniform throughout the body, trabecular bone being affected earlier and more severely than compact bone; this accounts for the disproportionate frequency of involvement of the distal radius, the neck of the femur and the vertebral bodies, all of which depend upon the integrity of trabecular bone.

Clinical presentation is according to the particular manifestation in the individual. In the case of back pain the pattern is helpful in making the diagnosis. Typically the pain is not present on waking, becomes worse through the day and is relieved by rest at night. The absence of stiffness is of assistance and there is preservation of movement in at least some planes. There is often accompanying osteoarthritis and degenerative disc disease with their separate distinguishable clinical contributions.

Various drugs or hormones in bewildering combinations are at present being recommended with equal enthusiasm by different authorities. These include:

1. Oestrogen alone. This suffers from its propensity to favour the development of endometrial neoplasia.
2. Oestrogen plus a progestational agent, which avoids the above problem but may be associated with an enhanced liability to coagulopathy.
3. Oestrogen +/− progestational agent together with active vitamin D.
4. The above together with fluoride. This may be associated with gastrointestinal upset and with soft tissue dystrophic calcification.
5. Calcitonin plus inorganic phosphate. This may be complicated by the development of an immune response and of allergy to the salmon polypeptide.
6. Diphosphonates. The complication of diphosphonate administration may be gastrointestinal in nature.
7. Anabolic steroids. There has been renewed interest in this possibility despite the fact that neither oestrogen nor androgen receptors have as yet been demonstrated in bone. The complications of anabolic steroids include masculinisation, fluid retention and the development of abnormal liver function tests.

A diet adequate in the provision of calcium and vitamin D is a prerequisite to all of these regimens. Again, the prophylactic value of regular exercise throughout life has been understated, the action of muscle activity on its bony insertions operating against the tendency towards loss of bone substance. The major therapeutic effect of most of these regimens lies in their ability to decrease the rate of loss of bone and only in the case of fluoride is it suggested that there may be an increase in bone formation. Even here the quality of the new bone laid down under the influence of fluoride with respect to its type of crystal formation has recently been questioned. The obvious corollary is that if anything is to be achieved then therapy must begin before there has been much bone loss and all the problems of instituting therapy in a group of people who at the time are virtually "normal" must be considered. For the immediate future we draw our reader's attention to this exciting and fast-developing field and recommend following it closely over the next few years. We reiterate our advice to focus attention upon general principles and well-tried preventive measures, in particular regular exercise, but we counsel caution for the moment from the point of view of active specific pharmacological intervention until more well-controlled studies have become available.

Paget's Disease

This is another condition in which our understanding of the underlying pathology is improving apace. Paget's disease becomes increasingly common with advancing years. Approximately 3% of persons in their fourth decade and over 11% of those in their eighth decade will have radiological evidence of this disease. Such figures must be interpreted in the context of an ageing population. Pathologically the hallmark is chaotic remodelling of bone in a scattered distribution, the sites of predilection being the spine, femora and pelvis and skull. The primary defect probably resides in the osteoclast, and the enhanced activity of the osteoblast is viewed as being compensatory. The cause of the defect is not yet fully understood but virus-like particles have been described recently in the cytoplasm of the osteoclast. It has been suggested by different workers that these may be either measles or rheovirus and that this is another example of a "slow virus" disease.

Biochemical indices of increased bone activity are a raised alkaline phosphatase level and increased hydroxyproline excretion. In a proportion of patients there may be elevated serum total, and ionisable, calcium, and in a few patients the serum concentration of parathormone is high. In some of these patients the high calcium concentrations may be a product of immobilisation but this is not the explanation in others. It seems that in most patients, despite the florid abnormalities which may include a twenty-fold increase in the turnover rate of calcium, the normal coupling mechanism linking deposition and removal is preserved. In a few patients who have the biochemical abnormalities in serum calcium and parathormone it seems that this coupling mechanism is disturbed. The characteristic radiological changes are well known and do not require emphasis.

Clinically the most common presentation is by accidental discovery on routine X-ray. Bone pain may be due to the disease or to its complications. These include deformity of the abnormal softened bone, fracture, secondary osteoarthritis or osteogenic sarcoma. Paget's disease is complicated by malignancy in approximately 2% of cases, and it is important to be aware of this although the incidence has been exaggerated in the past. Other complications include compression neuropathies and paraplegia. Deafness due to pressure on the auditory nerve and very rarely congestive cardiac failure may occur, although it is likely that the latter only happens in those patients in whom cardiac reserve is already severely compromised.

The disease tends to progress through a course of remissions and exacerbations and it is not uncommon for the process to enter a spontaneous and prolonged remission. Management must be individualised in accordance with serial assessments of symptoms, clinical signs and biochemical indices including alkaline phosphatase and urinary hydroxyproline concentrations.

Pain may be treated in the first instance by administration of the minimum dosage of the single most effective antirheumatic or analgesic drug selected on the basis of patient preference. The complications of the disease will require appropriate treatment in their own right and it is interesting that the rate of healing and of callus formation both in Paget's disease and in osteopenia is normal. The orthopaedic surgeons state that surgical intervention in Paget's disease is complicated not by delay in healing but by problems caused by the increased vascularity of the bone at operation.

There have been some interesting recent developments in the pharmacological management of Paget's disease. Calcitonin, diphosphonates and drugs such as mithramycin, a potent inhibitor of RNA synthesis which has a selective effect on actively dividing cells such as osteoclasts and which may also stimulate calcitonin production, are being examined.

Calcitonin

Calcitonin is a 32 amino acid polypeptide which has been sequenced and synthesised. Salmon, porcine and human hormone differ only by one or two amino acids but both porcine and salmon calcitonin are immunogenic in man. Allergic reactions may occur and antibody formation may interfere with the action of the hormone. It is administered by subcutaneous injection in units of 0.5 or 1 g for the human or in MRC units for the porcine or salmon material, in which the unit doses are 160 and 100 respectively. In the short-term, bone pain may be relieved in as short a time as 10 days to 2 weeks, and it is present practice to prescribe 6-month courses in a dose graduated in accordance with response. In patients with severe bone changes (in particular those with compression effects) treatment may require to be continued for as long as 2 years. Biochemical changes including a fall in alkaline phosphatase and a fall in urinary hydroxyproline concentrations occur early but in approximately 50% of patients there is a plateau effect in both clinical and biochemical response which is not due to antibody effect and which may be disappointing. The basis of this partial response is not at present understood. Adverse reactions include nausea, vomiting and diarrhoea, and pruritus.

Diphosphonates

These are analogues of pyrophosphate in which the P–O–P is replaced by P–C–P. Pyrophosphate is important in calcification and diphosphonates interfere with this process. They also inhibit nucleation and dissolution of hydroxyapatite crystals and retard both bone resorption and bone formation in animals. This has led to exploration of their usefulness in disorders associated with enhanced bone formation and deposition, such as Paget's disease and myositis ossificans. At the moment EHDP (dicalcium editronate disodium hydroxyethylate-1-2-diphosphonate) is available, but a profusion of other analogues are at various stages of preparation and will become available shortly. EHDP is administered orally although absorption is slow and incomplete and the dose is 20 mg/kg/day. EHDP produces a reduction in the numbers of osteoclasts and is effective in the treatment of Paget's disease. Symptomatic relief and changes in biochemical values occur within a few weeks of starting treatment. Adverse reactions which may be encountered include osteomalacia, and gastrointestinal symptoms which may be produced include dyspepsia and diarrhoea. Bone pain and fractures may occur and there may be a rise in serum alkaline phosphatase.

In an attempt to overcome the plateau effect of calcitonin, a combination of diphosphonate and calcitonin together is now being assessed.

The possibility of using mithramycin is being explored at present, but the prohibitive toxicity of this drug on liver, kidneys and platelets is a major problem.

Conclusion

Considerable advances have been made in our understanding of bone pathology and the pathogenesis of bone diseases and it is becoming more and more likely that we stand on the verge of equivalent advances in management. A great deal of information is becoming available and it is important that these proposed new therapeutic initiatives be assessed most rigorously. One of the major difficulties in gauging the effects of any treatment on bone is the time required for any effect which may be produced to become manifest and this also imposes the need for the most careful experimental design.

Further Reading

Boyle IT (1981) Osteoporosis. Scott Med J 26: 71–80
Brenton DP, Dent CE (1976) Idiopathic juvenile osteoporosis. In: Bickel H, Stem J (eds) Inborn errors of calcium and bone metabolism. MTP Press, Lancaster

Hamby RC (1981) Paget's disease of bone. Praeger Publishers, New York
Kanis JA (1976) Bone disease and calcitonin. Armour Pharmaceutical Co., Eastbourne
Kenzora JE, Glimcher MJ (1981) Osteonecrosis. In: Kelly W, Harris ED Jr, Ruddy S, Sledge CB
    (eds) Textbook of rheumatology, 1st edn. Saunders, Philadelphia London Toronto, Chap 108
Singer FR (1981) Metabolic bone disease. In: Kelly W, Harris ED Jr, Ruddy S, Sledge CB (eds)
    Textbook of rheumatology, 1st edn. Saunders, Philadelphia London Toronto, Chap 107
Sledge CB (1981) Formation and resorption of bone. In: Kelly W, Harris ED Jr, Ruddy S, Sledge
    CB (eds) Textbook of rheumatology, 1st edn. Saunders, Philadelphia London Toronto, Chap
    19
Vaughan J (1975) The physiology of bone. Clarendon, Oxford

6 Crystal Arthropathies

Introduction

A group of diseases, fast expanding, are marked by the deposition in tissue of crystals which appear to produce tissue destruction by a common mechanism. Either they are ingested by, or nucleation occurs within the cytoplasm of, polymorphonuclear leucocytes. There is abundant evidence that the white cell responds by trying to digest or destroy these crystals. The rate of all measured metabolic processes of these cells increases, neutral and acidic proteinases are formed within the primary and secondary lysosomes of these cells and these and other products of the cells leak into the extracellular fluid, reducing the local pH. Potentially toxic products of oxygen metabolism and products of cell membrane lysis such as prostaglandins, leukotrienes, interleukins and superoxides are released and an acute inflammatory reaction ensues which may limit or promote further destruction according to local circumstances. In the past individual crystals have been linked to different diseases. Recently it has been appreciated that the position may be considerably more complex.

It is important to understand the process by which crystals are formed in vivo. Too little attention has been paid to the natural inhibitors of crystal deposition. For example serum albumin and tissue proteins bind urate and inhibit nucleation and the divalent cation magnesium opposes nucleation of calcium pyrophosphate crystals, the opposite being true for high concentrations of calcium or iron. These effects are the explanation for some of the disease associations which have been documented, such as the relationships between haemochromatosis, hypercalcaemic states or hypomagnesaemia and calcium pyrophosphate crystal deposition disease (CPPD). It is also important to be aware of the phenomenon termed "epitaxy". This expresses the enhancement of nucleation of one crystal in the presence of another which has already undergone the process of nucleation. The implication of this in the clinic will be increased recognition of clinical states associated with not one, but with an array of different crystals.

Gout

This was well known to Hippocrates, who noted that it was rare in prepubertal males, in eunuchs and in women before the menopause. An acute attack of gouty arthritis, "podagra", is one of the most classical clinical cameos and has been a source of mirth and distress throughout the ages. This is only one of the consequences of hyperuricaemia, which may be the result either of enhanced production or of impaired excretion of uric acid (Fig. 6.1). A diagrammatic

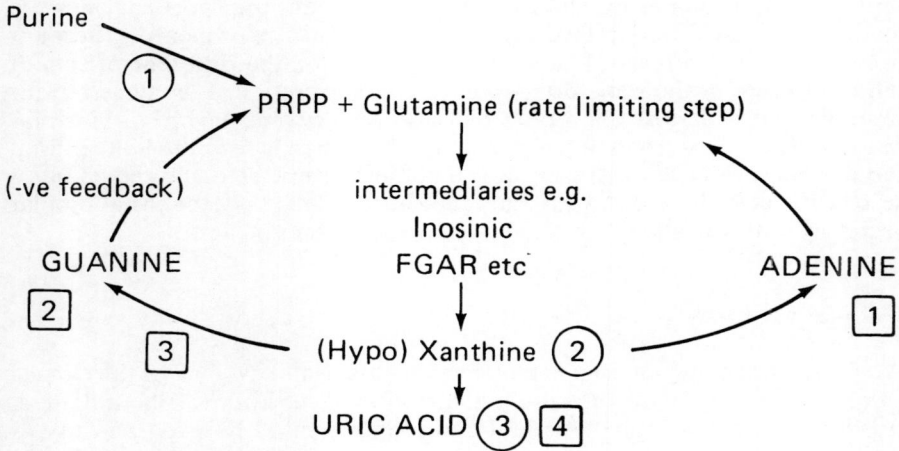

ENZYME DEFECTS

1 Adenine deaminases

2 Guanine phosphorylases (both produce selective immuno-deficiency)

3 HGPRT (hypoxanthine guanine phosphoribosyl transferase)

4 ? defect in transport or urate across renal tubule

SITES OF INTERACTION WITH DRUGS

1 Treatment of malignancy with cytotoxic drugs

2 Allopurinol (oxypurinol)

3 Organic anions e.g. diuretics, NSAID etc

    ACETYLSALICYLIC ACID   high doses reduce serum uric acid
                                   produce uricosuria

                       low doses raise serum uric acid
                               reduce urine uric acid

Fig. 6.1. Purine biosynthetic pathways (abbreviated)

representation of the de novo purine biosynthetic pathway is provided upon which are recorded the important enzyme deficiencies and the sites of interaction with various drugs. It is noteworthy that the diseases involved have been expanded recently to include a group of selective immunodeficiencies.

Homo sapiens, by some evolutionary twist, has lost the enzyme uricase which catalyses the further metabolism of uric acid to allantoin. Uric acid therefore has become the final product of this pathway and must be excreted by the kidney. It is thought that this is accomplished in the following manner: urate is filtered completely at the glomerulus and all of the filtered urate is reabsorbed in the proximal tubule. The uric acid which appears in the urine represents secretion at the distal tubule and different transport enzymes are involved at these different levels. This is the explanation proposed to account for the different effects of different drugs and for the different effects of different doses of the same drug upon uric acid excretion. It is suggested for example that high doses of aspirin block all the enzymes involved. Since far more urate is reabsorbed in the proximal tubule than is secreted by the distal tubular enzyme systems, the result is a net loss of uric acid and reduction of serum uric acid. Low doses, on the other hand, block only the distal tubular secretory pathway and produce an increase in serum uric acid.

Clinical Features

An acute attack of gout is an explosive event associated with all of the clinical local and systemic signs of acute inflammation. The skin over the inflamed, swollen, and excruciatingly painful and tender joint is hot, red and dry as opposed to the skin overlying a septic lesion, which is moist. The stick held in the hand of the gouty patient is not to assist walking but to fend off intruders. The pain is so severe that the patient cannot tolerate another person even in the immediate vicinity. Evidence of constitutional involvement includes pyrexia, polymorphonuclear leucocytosis and a rise in the acute phase proteins. Although many patients experience only a single episode throughout their entire lives, others may develop chronic tophaceous gout and nephrolithiasis without ever passing through the stage of acute gout. The kidneys are very rarely involved in the absence of articular disease. The joint most frequently involved in the first and in subsequent episodes is the first metatarsophalangeal joint; thereafter the knee, ankle, wrist and the small joints of the hands and feet may be affected. A small proportion of patients experience a polyarticular pattern.

Chronic tophaceous gout produces a different type of pain of a less acute nature. The patient complains of a dull aching pain with associated stiffness and swelling of the small joints of the hands and feet which may add to the similarity to rheumatoid arthritis. However, the pattern is usually less symmetrical in evolution and distribution. Tophaceous deposits should be sought in avascular areas such as the pinnae of the ears, in relationship to tendons and joints and in particular in exposed extensor surfaces of the limbs. Rarely they may occur in almost any visceral site. These tophi may cause trouble by local pressure or simply because of their position. They may rupture through the skin, extruding chalky pultaceous material, and may form a chronic sinus. Whether after spontaneous rupture or after elective surgery, the resultant wound may prove to be very slow to heal.

The following may be associated with gout:

Obesity/starvation diets	Diabetes mellitus
Hypertension	Hyperlipidaemia
Atherosclerosis	Renal impairment
CPPD	Nephrolithiasis
Chronic meloid leukaemia	Polycythaemia rubra vera
HGPRTG-b-PD deficiency	Drugs (including alcohol)[1]

It is interesting that there are wide differences throughout the world in the prevalence of both hyperuricaemia and gout. In the Maori in New Zealand approximately 40% of the adult male population are hyperuricaemic and as many as 10% have clinical gout. Even within the United Kingdom gout is more common in the north-east than it is either south of this in London or north in the west of Scotland. It is likely that serum uric acid is under a combination of environmental and polygenic influences. Certainly it is worth taking a family history carefully from the patient; this should include the direct manifestations of hyperuricaemia and all associated and co-diseases.

The other organ which bears the brunt of hyperuricaemia is the kidney. Pathologically the kidney in patients with gout may show signs of associated or complicating diseases such as hypertensive changes. There may be an interstitial nephritis but the hallmark of the gouty kidney is crystal deposition. In the tubules uric acid itself may be precipitated, producing anuria and a medical emergency; whilst this is rare, cancer treatment with cytotoxic drugs may lead to a massive uric acid load on the kidney. More commonly monosodium urate is deposited in the interstitium. It should be remembered that the kidney may be affected by the drugs used to treat the disease, and the NSAIDs are the most obvious examples of this. The long continued use of these prostaglandin synthetase inhibitors may affect renal function adversely.

Drug Treatment

Whereas with most of the other rheumatic disorders it is most important to explore fully all the possibilities of non-drug treatment, mainly because the drugs available are both toxic and of limited efficacy, here the primary step in management is the selection and proper prescription of highly effective drugs.

In patients with acute gout the drug of choice is indomethacin and if that is not appropriate then naproxen or one of the other non-steroidal drugs will control the acute attack. There is now no role for phenylbutazone—not because it is ineffective (indeed, on the contrary, it was a very effective drug)

---

1. Increasingly diuretic therapy, often ill-advised, is becoming the most common cause of hyperuricaemia and gout.

but because there are so many equally effective and less toxic alternatives. Whichever of the first line drugs is selected it is important that it be prescribed properly and this can be illustrated best in the context of indomethacin. The first step is to appreciate the pain that the patient is suffering and to aim for the most prompt relief. A large loading dose of the drug should be administered as soon as possible. The speed and completeness of response is dictated largely by how early in the evolution of the condition effective treatment is prescribed. It is interesting in this context how seldom today we encounter patients with "resistant" acute gout compared with only 15–20 years ago and this is in large measure because effective treatment is being instituted at a far earlier stage, very often by the patient's own general practitioner. Account must be taken of the patient's age, sex and especially their weight. It is also interesting how seldom the very same side-effects which can be so troublesome in other patients with different diseases requiring more long-term treatment are encountered in this context. Certainly even normal subjects exposed to the same dose of indomethacin acutely will experience the most miserable side-effects at this dose level, as each of the authors can testify to personally. In acute gout it is as if there was an "inflammatory sump" into which the drug was absorbed, leaving little free drug to produce adverse reactions. It has to be stated that there is no evidence whatsoever to support this proposition at the moment. However, it is also important to note that as soon as the patient begins to feel relief then the dose must be reduced promptly because it is at this stage that the patient may begin to experience adverse reactions. A similar situation obtains in the treatment of very acute SLE with prednisolone. Again, the drug is well tolerated in high dose during periods of the most active inflammation and again side-effects appear as soon as the activity of the disease begins to decline.

Although of mainly historical interest, it is worth spending a moment on colchicine. This used to be obtained from the autumn crocus and has a long and distinguished history dating back to the sixth century A.D. It is rapidly absorbed from the gastrointestinal tract and is excreted in bile and urine. The plasma half-life is of the order of 20 min. Side-effects commonly encountered include severe dyspepsia and diarrhoea, and if colchicine is given intravenously it may produce very severe local inflammation and even tissue necrosis. Colchicine produces an interesting inhibitory effect on the intracellular microtubules at a concentration which leaves the microfilaments relatively unscathed, and it will stop the cell cycle in metaphase. These effects are of particular interest in the laboratory but because of these properties it is possible that colchicine may find a role in diseases other than gout. The recent work on the amyloidosis secondary to familial mediterranean fever is a case in point.

The other clinical situation in which indomethacin, another first line antirheumatic drug, or colchicine may be used in this context is as a prophylactic against the development of an acute attack during the institution of interval treatment of gout or of marked hyperuricaemia. In this case smaller doses are adequate.

Chronic Tophaceous Gout

This should now be an anachronism residing more in the slide boxes of aged lecturers than in the clinic. Certainly rare cases are still seen, but it is important in these patients to look more deeply for the primary diagnosis, which is non-compliance for one of many possible reasons. Many of the patients in this category seen today are alcoholic, of low intelligence or mentally ill. This dramatic reversal of fortunes is attributable to the recent availability of highly effective and in one case specific drug therapy.

The uricosuric drugs became available first. Probenecid arose from a compound which was initially developed to block the excretion of penicillin by the renal tubular cell and hence to enhance its bioavailability. Since there is a common tubular mechanism which serves the purpose of transporting organic anions, it was hardly surprising that it also blocked the renal transport across the tubular cell of another organic anion, urate. The reason that the result of blocking the bidirectional pathway causes a net increase in the rate of elimination of the anion is that far greater quantities are reabsorbed initially by the proximal tubule than are secreted later by the distal tubule.

Probenecid is completely absorbed by the gastrointestinal tract in 2–4 h and has a plasma half-life of 6–12 h. It is excreted in alkaline but not in acid urine and is not bound to plasma proteins. It is metabolised in the hepatocyte to form a glucuronide, a hydroxylate and a carboxylate, the latter two being themselves uricosuric. The dose is of the order of 0.5–1.5 g per day. In a dose of 20 mg/kg probenecid will produce a four-fold increase in urinary uric acid output promptly.

Sulphinpyrazone was discovered by adjustment of the phenylbutazone molecule when it was found to have a uricosuric effect. It is completely absorbed within 2 h and has a half-life of 3 h. It is strongly bound to plasma proteins and secreted by the renal tubules. Its metabolite, p-hydroxysulphin-pyrazole, is uricosuric, and the drug is more effective on a weight-for-weight basis than probenecid. The daily dose is 300–400 mg.

Probenecid and sulphinpyrazone act by a similar mechanism and both will block the non-specific renal tubular anion transport mechanism. Thus they will also interfere with the transport of penicillin, serotonin, dopamine, cortico-trophin and cAMP.

Adverse reactions which are common to both include gastrointestinal upset and the development of hypersensitivity reactions. With both there is a risk of renal urate nephrolithiasis and of the development of acute gout during the early stages of treatment, as is also the case with allopurinol. This last effect is probably related to wide fluctuations which occur in local tissues when hitherto stable deposits of urate are mobilised. Probenecid will increase the renal elimination of allopurinol when these drugs are prescribed together. Sulphinpyrazone may produce marrow depression and exerts a significant effect on platelet aggregation. Azapropazone, an anti-inflammatory drug, has uricosuric properties and may prove to be of value in acute and chronic gout.

Allopurinol is now the drug of choice for all patients with hyperuricaemia or any of its consequences when drug therapy is required. Allopurinol [4-hydroxypyrazolo-(3,4-d) pyrimidine] is a structural isomer of hypoxanthine and a competitive inhibitor of xanthine oxidase (Fig. 6.1). It is metabolised to a dihydroxy metabolite, oxypurinol, which also possesses this action and which has a longer half-life in the body. From the table it is obvious that inhibition at that site will reduce the concentration of subsequent products and will increase the amount of the precursors xanthine and hypoxanthine. Fortunately these are both much more soluble than is uric acid and the complication of treatment which might have been expected to be a problem, namely xanthine crystalluria, is not common and is only encountered in patients with congenital xanthinuria or the Lesch-Nyhan syndrome. Allopurinol also exerts a further effect on the purine biosynthetic pathway. In the presence of HGPRT when allopurinol blocks the further metabolism of xanthine and hypoxanthine, hypoxanthine finds its easiest further metabolic pathway in conversion to the purines guanine and adenine. The rise in concentration of these purines itself exerts a negative feedback inhibition on the rate-limiting enzymic reaction and inhibits the de novo purine biosynthetic pathway.

Allopurinol is well absorbed from the gastrointestinal tract, peak plasma levels occurring in 2–6 h and the plasma half-life is of the order of 2–3 h. The dihydroxy metabolite formed in the hepatocyte, oxypurinol, has a half-life of 20–30 h and is handled by the renal tubule in a manner similar to uric acid. This is why urate clearance is increased by the simultaneous prescription of uricosuric drugs. After continuous administration an equilibrium effect is reached in 2–4 days. Serum uric acid begins to fall 24–48 h after therapy is initiated.

In addition to treatment of established gout and nephrolithiasis, allopurinol may also be used prophylactically in clinical situations where it is desired to reduce dangerously high serum uric acid concentrations, for example in the management of malignancy with cytotoxic drugs. The dose is of the order of 300 mg to 1.2 g per day. In the first few weeks of treatment it is necessary to provide the patient with a prophylactic antirheumatic drug, so common is the precipitation of acute gouty arthritis during this time. In fact, despite the occasional dyspepsia or skin rash, the only significant adverse reaction encountered with allopurinol is acute gout. The response to allopurinol is so predictable and so complete that patients labelled "failed allopurinol" should be thoroughly investigated to exclude another possible diagnosis or non-compliance. Failing this, the next most common cause of lack of response is inadequate dosage.

Once started, treatment may have to be continued for life, which makes the initial decision to start so important. Since a considerable number of patients experience only one episode of gout throughout their entire life it is unwise to make this decision on the basis of a single episode. Hyperuricaemia alone is rarely a sufficient indication to start treatment except in the particular instance of treatment of malignancy with cytotoxic drugs or in the presence of very high serum concentrations.

The only other factor of importance to discuss in the context of allopurinol is the very rare occurrence of depression of marrow elements or the precipitation of vasculitis in a manner analogous to the thiazides. Allopurinol will interfere with other drugs which involve xanthine oxidase in their metabolism. Thus it will potentiate the effect and the adverse reactions of 6-mercaptopurine and azathioprine on bone marrow.

Calcium Pyrophosphate Crystal Deposition Disease (CPPD)

The deposition of CPPD in tissue can produce a variety of clinical syndromes. Although the presentation of a red hot joint ("pseudogout") has been emphasised, this is in fact the least common manifestation. More commonly the patient masquerades in the routine clinic with the label "osteoarthritis" until someone recognises either that the patient is pursuing a course characterised by more acute exacerbations than usual or that X-ray reveals chondrocalcinosis.

Diagnostic criteria for CPPD are:

1. Demonstration of CaPPi crystals (obtained by biopsy, necropsy or aspiration and identified definitively, e.g. X-ray diffraction powder pattern or "finger-print")
2. Demonstration of mono- or tri-clinic crystals with no or only weakly positively birefringent behaviour on compensated polarising microscopy
3. Presence of *typical* calcification on X-ray
4. Acute episodes of arthritis (especially large joints, e.g. knee)
5. Chronic arthritis, especially of knee or hip and especially associated with acute exacerbations

For a definite diagnosis to be made, items 1, 2 and 3 must be present; if 2 and 3 are present, diagnosis will be "probable". Items 4 and 5 should alert the clinician to the possibility of CPPD.

Calcium pyrophosphate is found commonly in the joints of elderly patients at routine postmortems. The most common age of onset lies in the sixth or seventh decade, few cases occurring under the age of 40. In this country most cases are sporadic but well-documented instances of a familial pattern have been published. Very recently a metabolic defect in such families has been defined. In these patients the age of onset tends to be younger and the arthritis is more severe. The following four clinical patterns have been described.

Pseudogout

This is the "red hot joint". The attack differs from gout in that onset is less abrupt and the attack is less severe and less disabling. The attack may last from as short a period as 1 day to a prolonged episode lasting for up to 4–6 weeks. Sometimes the condition may begin in one joint and then spread to involve other joints to form "cluster" attacks. The knees and then the wrist joints are most commonly involved, but other joints, including the first metatarsophalangeal joint, are not exempt.

Pseudorheumatoid Disease

Multiple subacute joint involvement may produce a clinical picture very similar to rheumatoid arthritis and the confusion may be compounded by the accompaniment of other features such as morning stiffness and "gelling", fatigue and malaise, and an elevated ESR. Usually there is less symmetry, less evidence of a major proliferative component and absence of the extra-articular complications of rheumatoid arthritis. Furthermore, nodules are absent and rheumatoid factor is not present in significant titre. Very rarely "classical" rheumatoid arthritis and CPPD may coexist, in which case it is necessary to adduce all of the evidence required to make each diagnosis independently. The other situation in which rheumatoid arthritis or indeed almost any disease which produces articular damage may interact with CPPD is when pyrophosphate crystals are found in the synovial fluid of a patient who in all other respects is suffering only from "classical" rheumatoid arthritis. This is an important observation which has only been made recently and it raises the question of whether the crystal causes the disease or the disease and damage to the joint create the local circumstances which favour the process of nucleation and crystal growth.

Pseudo-osteoarthritis

It is now perfectly obvious that "osteoarthritis" is a name applicable only to a syndrome which may be produced by a variety of different mechanisms. Any of the crystal deposition diseases may be a factor in the production of this syndrome, and CPPD is no exception. Pseudo-osteoarthritis occurs most commonly in elderly females and the knee, wrist, metacarpophalangeal, hip, shoulders, elbows and ankles are involved in decreasing order. Often the only clinical clues are the presence of unexpectedly abrupt and severe exacerbations and of more joint destruction than usual. The site of involvement may be of assistance since it is so uncommon for the wrist, shoulder or elbow to be involved in uncomplicated osteoarthritis.

Pseudoneuropathic Joint (Charcot's Joint)

Charcot's joint is the term applied to indicate a joint which is the seat of a conspicuously destructive disease process. It is often said that these are painless but this is certainly not a reliable clinical marker. Originally, the disease described in association with this clinical state was the "poor man's" expression of neurosyphilis, namely taboparesis. Today, in the lower limbs the more likely cause is diabetes. In the upper limb an additional possibility is syringomyelia. Other causes include repeated intra-articular injection of corticosteroid, infection and congenital insensitivity to pain. The radiological picture may mimic leprosy. In a similar manner to that described above, calcium pyrophosphate crystals have been found in Charcot's joints and the same question of cause and effect applies.

Treatment

Diseases which may be associated with CPPD include:

Haemochromatosis/haemosiderosis + Wilson's disease

Hyperparathyroidism (and other hypercalcaemic states)

Hyperuricaemia and gout

Hyperglycaemia and diabetes mellitus

Hypophosphatasia

Homogentisic acid oxidase deficiency (ochronosis)

Hypothyroidism

Hypermobility

The treatment of CPPD is entirely empirical and therefore differs markedly from the treatment of gout. Again, therefore, the emphasis must be upon general methods of management and non-pharmacological intervention techniques (Chaps. 2, 3, 13).

The best approach to an acute episode is a combination of the single most effective and least toxic first-line drug selected on the basis of patient preference in the first instance, followed if necessary by joint aspiration and lavage. In the event of failure of response to these measures one or at the most two injections of corticosteroid injected intra-articularly may be effective. Aspiration of synovial fluid provides material for crystal identification and as always a sample must be sent to the bacteriological laboratory. The acutely inflamed joint must be rested, if necessary with the aid of a splint. It is very important to ensure that the joint is splinted in the correct position. Management of the subacute and chronic patient embraces all of the general measures and pharmacological principles described above. The indications for surgical intervention are defined above and the importance of individualised management of the patient and of the need for an active aggressive and supportive programme of rehabilitation need no further emphasis, nor does the need to identify and treat complicating and co-diseases.

Calcium Apatite

Calcium hydroxyapatite is one of the important structural crystals of bone. Recently it has been recognised that these crystals may also occur in joints and in soft tissues. The delay in appreciating this is in part attributable to the difficulty of identifying these crystals. The techniques of scanning and transmission electron microscopy and X-ray diffraction are required whereas urate and calcium pyrophosphate crystals may be visualised by light microscopy and identified by the manner in which they rotate polarised light.

The deposition of calcium apatite may be involved in different clinical situations. An acute subacromial bursitis or perhaps a capsulitis of shoulder may be produced in this way. In the former there may be X-ray evidence of calcification but this is often present in shoulders which are not clinically inflamed, indicating that there must be an additional local factor involved. Patients with uraemia may develop widespread deposition of calcium apatite throughout soft tissues in many parts of the body. Recently these crystals have been identified in the joints of some patients with "osteoarthritis" and the considerations referred to above apply. The patients in whom these crystals have been seen are particularly prone to experience acute inflammatory episodes, synovial effusions, morning stiffness and "gelling" and "hot" Heberden's nodes. Treatment of these patients is as for those with CPPD.

Further Reading

Abramson S, Hoffstein ST, Weissman G (1982) Superoxide anion generation by human neutrophils exposed to monosodium urate. Arthritis Rheum 25: 174–180

Dieppe PA (1978) Crystal arthritis. In: Dick WC, Buchanan WW (eds) Recent advances in rheumatology, 2nd edn. Churchill Livingstone, Edinburgh London New York

Dieppe PA, Calvert PR (in press) A practical guide to polarising light microscopy. In: Dieppe PA, Calvert PR (eds) Crystal induced arthritis and related diseases. Chapman and Hall, London

Dieppe PA, Crocker PR, Corke CF, Doyle DV, Huskisson EC, Willoughby DA (1979) Synovial fluid crystals. J Med, New Series XLVIII (192): 533–553

Fessel WJ (1972) Hyperuricaemia in health and disease. Semin Arthritis Rheum 1: 275–299

Hesselbacher P (1979) C3 activation by monosodium urate monohydrate and other crystalline material. Arthritis Rheum 22: 571–578

Howell DS (1981) Diseases due to the deposition of calcium pyrophosphate and hydroxyapatite. In: Kelly W, Harris ED Jr, Ruddy S, Sledge CB (eds) Textbook of rheumatology, 1st edn. Saunders, Philadelphia London Toronto, Chap 87

Kelly WN (1981) Gout and related disorders of purine metabolism. In: Kelly W, Harris ED Jr, Ruddy S, Sledge CB (eds) Textbook of rheumatology, 1st edn. Saunders, Philadelphia London Toronto, Chap 86

McCarty DJ Jr, Hogan JM, Gatter RE, Grossman M (1966) Studies on pathological calcifications in human cartilage. J Bone Joint Surg 48A(2): 309–325

McGuire MKB, Hearn PR, Russell RCG (1980) Calcium pyrophosphate crystals (their relevance to C.P.P.D., pseudogout, chondrocalcinosis and pyrophosphate arthropathy); biochemical and physicochemical aspects. In: Maroudas A, Hoborrow EJ (eds) Studies in joint disease—1. Pitman Medical, Tunbridge Wells, pp 117–156

7 General Medical and Metabolic Diseases

Haemophilia

Both haemophilia A (factor VIII) and haemophilia B (factor IX) are inherited as X-linked recessive diseases and in both the functional defect is in the intrinsic pathway, the extrinsic tissue-factor-dependent pathway being the only mechanism left intact to subserve haemostasis. The most important consequence of haemophilia is arthritis and it is interesting that synovial tissue is deficient in tissue factor, which may explain this association. Arthritis occurs only in those patients who are severely affected, with concentrations of circulating antihaemophiliac globulin of less than 5%, and onset is usually in childhood. The knee and the elbow joints are most commonly involved and may become swollen acutely either spontaneously or after only the most minor trauma. Range of movement, usually preserved after the first episode, is progressively lost with subsequent attacks and severe joint destruction and deformity may follow. Extra-articular bleeding is also common.

Pathologically there is a chronic proliferative non-specific synovitis with extensive haemosiderin deposition and fibrosis. Haemorrhages occur both into the joint and in subchondral bone. Radiologically soft tissue swelling proceeds to local osteopenia, the development of large subchondral and juxta-articular bone cysts, cartilage destruction and secondary osteoarthritis. Fibrous bony ankylosis may follow but true bony ankylosis is uncommon.

The diagnosis is usually perfectly straightforward and frequently will have been made in the past. The usual presentation is a child with a single swollen peripheral joint. The most troublesome differential diagnosis is from infection and the haemophiliac joint is itself at risk from this complication. The other group of conditions which may be confused with this presentation in this age group is juvenile chronic arthritis. Bleeding into muscles and non-articular soft tissues may be the presenting complaint. Bleeding into the forearm may produce Volkmann's ischaemic contracture, into the gastrocnemius a talipes equinus deformity, and into the iliopsoas a flexed hip with pain in the groin. The last may be distinguished from an intra-articular process in the normal classical way by demonstrating that passive rotation of the hip is preserved. Once suspected, the diagnosis is confirmed by demonstration of the specific coagulopathy. The family history may of course provide the diagnostic clue and may permit initiation of treatment in hitherto unaffected children at the earliest possible moment.

The limiting factor in treatment is prompt diagnosis, both initially and with each successive bleeding episode, and the recent improvement in prognosis represents a synthesis of prompt recognition coupled with the immediate institution of effective treatment. Home programmes incorporating prophylaxis have contributed in large measure to the improved prognosis. Severely affected patients will require replacement as often as weekly at some stages in their disease, and it is particularly important in such patients that their requirements are properly calculated and that circulating anti-factor VIII or IX antibodies are detected if present. It seems that there may be a familial predisposition to the development of these acquired inhibitors.

The aim, therefore, is prevention rather than treatment, and the combination of specialty hospital units working together with the family doctor and an informed family has improved the outlook for these children dramatically. The most important adverse reaction to cryoprecipitate or factor concentrates apart from allergic reactions is hepatitis, which may be of the A, B or non-A, non-B variety. The indications for elective surgical intervention in those patients who do not possess inhibitor antibodies are in accord with general principles and the management of local articular or extra-articular bleeding likewise should follow routine lines. Once bleeding has been controlled by the prompt elevation of the circulating factor concentration to at least 50% of normal then there may be a case for aspiration of a haemarthrosis. The presence of blood in the articular cavity is all that is required to produce the histopathological abnormalities of the disease in dogs. The importance of maintaining local muscle power and tone around an affected joint and of avoiding the development of a flexion deformity needs no further emphasis. The management of those unfortunate children who do develop circulating antibodies may tax the resources of the best team and is an area which only the specialist should direct.

Haemoglobinopathies

Arthritis and musculoskeletal complications occur commonly in patients with haemoglobinopathies. Many of these manifestations are common to the process of chronic haemolysis rather than to the underlying specific metabolic defect. In all there is a tendency to marrow expansion with trabecular changes in the axial skeleton, and in HbS this process extends to the peripheral long bones and even to the phalanges, producing the "hand-foot" syndrome which may be the presenting complaint. The extremities are inflamed and swollen and the child may be toxic and pyrexial. Other features which may be common to several of the haemoglobinopathies include avascular necrosis of bone and bone infarction, peripheral synovitis with effusions, hyperuricaemia and rarely gout, and an arthropathy associated with secondary haemochromatosis. Some complications are related more specifically to individual defects such as the relationships between (a) osteomyelitis (especially with salmonellae) of the hip and sickle cell disease or (b) arthritis of the ankle and osteomalacia with thalassaemia. Sickle cell disease and most of the others are diseases of amino-acid substitution whereas thalassaemia is a disorder of chain assembly. Treatment requires medical management of the haematological disorder together with special attention to the articular problems.

Myeloma

Musculoskeletal manifestations are frequently associated with myeloma and often occur as the presenting complaint. Back pain, polymyalgia rheumatica, hyperuricaemia and gout and a symmetrical inflammatory polyarthritis may all presage myeloma, but since these are all very common complaints the continual difficulty is to recognise the "signal" from the "noise". Very rarely myeloma may be associated with an oligoarthritis, often involving the shoulder joint, when there is profuse synovial proliferation and infiltration with amyloid.

Musculoskeletal manifestations are encountered commonly in other malignancies, ranging from the confusion at presentation in the child between leukaemia and JCP to the presence of an effusive, usually non-destructive polyarthritis in adults with solid tissue tumours.

Hypogammaglobulinaemia

Whether of the congenital or acquired variety, this is frequently associated with an inflammatory polyarthritis. Recent evidence linking immunodeficiency syndromes with genetically determined inborn errors in the purine biosynthetic pathway offers an exciting new prospect in our understanding of these diseases and may provide clues to the control of lymphocyte physiology.

Other Genetically Determined Inborn Errors of Metabolism

Arthritis and musculoskeletal manifestations occupy a more or less important place in the clinical features of a wide variety of diseases, alkaptonuria, Wilson's disease, homocystinuria, hyperlysinaemia, glycogen storage diseases and the mucopolysaccharidoses being obvious examples (see Chap. 2). The important point to make in a text of this nature is that the clinician must remain alert and must be prepared at all times to be confronted with such a circumstance. It may occur only seldom in the lifetime of any individual physician, yet the consequence to the patient may be considerable. The best rule is to question at all times the diagnosis in patients who present with multisystem involvement and in patients in whom the present diagnostic label does not quite fit.

The Hyperlipidaemias

The WHO classification of these interesting diseases is reproduced in Table 7.1 and the musculoskeletal complications which may be encountered in each are included in the table. Cystic lesions of bone may occur both in types 1 and 5 as well as in type 4. In type 2a, both in the homozygous and in the heterozygous patient, an acute migratory polyarthritis or periarthritis may be the presenting complaint and may allow early recognition and the institution of dietary and pharmacological control at a stage where prophylaxis has some hope of success; a similar although distinctive polyarthritis may complicate type 4 disease. Hyperuricaemia and gout may complicate or may occur as co-diseases in types 2 and 4, and tuberous and cutaneous xanthomas and xanthelasmata mark the presence of type 2 disease.

Table 7.1. The hyperlipidaemias (normal)

Type[a]	Lipoprotein E/P	Cholesterol	T/G	Inheritance	Xanthomata
1	Chylomicra	↑	↑ ↑	Auto. rec.	Eruptive
2 a)	Beta[a]	↑ ↑ ↑	n/ ↑	Auto. dom.	Arcus
b)	Beta and pre-beta[a]	↑ ↑ ↑	n/ ↑	Auto. dom.	Tendinous/ tuberous
3	Broad beta	↑ ↑	↑ ↑	Auto. rec.	Tendinous/ tubero-eruptive/ arcus
4	Pre-beta[a]	n	↑ ↑	Auto. dom.	Eruptive
5	Pre-beta/ chylomicra[a]	↑ ↑ ↑ ↑		Auto. dom.	Eruptive

[a] In types 2 and 4 there may be a migratory inflammatory polyarthritis. Hyperuricaemia and gout may complicate type 2, 4 and 5 disease.

The diseases associated with disorders of structural protein are covered in Chap. 2 and the lysosomal storage diseases are referred to in Table 2.2 in that chapter. Amyloidosis, a metabolic process which is at last yielding some of its secrets, is discussed in Chap. 8. Deposition of amyloid represents a combination of a contribution from elevated serum concentrations of precursors which may be acute phase proteins, hormones or segments of immunoglobulin molecules together with a local tissue product.

Haemochromatosis

In primary haemochromatosis most patients do not present until the fifth or sixth decade but it seems likely that there is a major genetic component. Linkage in over 76% of patients with HLA-A3 but in only 30% with HLA-B14 suggests that the gene responsible lies closer to the HLA-A locus. The data favour a recessive mode of inheritance. The underlying defect has not yet been defined, but an abnormal increase in the intestinal absorption of iron seems to be common to most patients.

There is an increase in uptake of iron by the hepatocyte, and transferrin, the iron transport protein, is saturated early. Ferritin, apoferritin, and reticuloendothelial iron are all increased and the concentration of the insoluble storage form of iron, namely haemosiderin, is increased.

The arthropathy associated with this has many of the features of severe osteoarthritis with superadded CPPD. The second and third metacarpophalangeal joints of the hand are involved conspicuously, alerting the clinician to the presence of an unusual variety of osteoarthritis, and acute inflammatory episodes should likewise draw attention to the underlying disease. The presence of chondrocalcinosis and the features of the systemic disease, including cirrhosis, slate-grey discolouration of the skin, diabetes, hypopituitarism and hypogonadism, lead to the diagnosis, which may be confirmed by demonstration of a reduced total iron binding capacity, elevated serum iron, transferrin saturation and in the later stages elevated serum ferritin. The definitive investigation is the demonstration of excessive iron on a quantitative basis in liver parenchyma.

Removal of excess iron does not necessarily improve the arthropathy, so management represents a combination of the general medical treatment of haemochromatosis coupled with the general principles of management of any chronic arthropathy.

Multicentric Histiocytosis

Although very rare, this disease, which probably represents an as yet uncharacterised storage and metabolic disease, presents in a manner which does draw attention to a clinical picture with an interesting differential diagnosis. The clinical picture is that of a patient with a chronic seronegative polyarthritis associated with subcutaneous nodule formation, and the conditions which may present in this way are listed in Table 7.2. Recent evidence has focussed attention upon this disease as a disturbance in the function of antigen-presenting, Birbeck granule-containing Langerhans' cells in skin.

Table 7.2. Polyarthritis associated with subcutaneous nodules in a seronegative patient

Metabolic diseases—gout, crystal deposition diseases, hyperlipoproteinaemias, amyloidosis
Rheumatic fever
Granuloma annulare
Multicentric reticulohistiocytosis
Juvenile chronic polyarthritis
Rheumatoid arthritis following treatment with second line drugs
Laboratory or transcription error
"Hidden rheumatoid factor" (RF flooded by excess non-specific immunoglobulins)

Arthritis Associated with Endocrine Diseases

As is the case in the diseases described above, one of the most important aspects of arthritis associated with other medical diseases is the opportunity that this combination may present to the clinician for early diagnosis. If this can lead to earlier institution of effective therapy then this is a point of considerable importance.

Diabetes Mellitus

It is now becoming more and more obvious that, like osteoarthritis, this term merely describes an end stage which may be the result of several different causes. The HLA associations of type 1 diabetes are of considerable interest to the rheumatologist and may teach us a great deal. It is of particular interest that the metabolic derangement in type 2 disease, which extends far beyond the boundaries of glucose handling, is itself marked by a genetic component of considerable magnitude.

A variety of musculoskeletal manifestations may be associated with diabetes mellitus—some as complications and some as co-diseases. Osteoarthritis of the knees and the lumbar spine is a common finding in patients with maturity onset diabetes although the association may be related more closely to the accompanying metabolic obesity. CPPD disease is associated with diabetes and the relationship is bidirectional. Diabetic osteolysis describes a syndrome in which there is florid osteopenia (usually in the bones of the foot), which may occur in the absence of a demonstrable neuropathy or vascular impairment and which may progress to collapse of the articular surface and a picture indistinguishable from a Charcot's joint. Septic arthritis and a true Charcot's neuropathic joint are well described (and require no emphasis), as are Forrestier's disease, carpal tunnel syndrome and Dupuytren's contracture. In the case of the last-mentioned there is a bidirectional association and the position is confused by the presence, even in young diabetic children, of palmar fascial disease and joint hypomobility. It is possible that a similar mechanism is responsible for the periarthritis of shoulder which is common in diabetics, and it has been suggested that post-translational glycosylation of tissue structural protein may be responsible for these connective tissue abnormalities.

Adrenal Disease

Cushing's syndrome, whether iatrogenic or spontaneously acquired, is associated with osteopenia and vertebral collapse, and it is insufficiently emphasised that this may occur after only a brief exposure to high dose corticosteroid therapy or to long-term low dose administration of prednisolone (less than 7.5 mg per day), underlining the importance of viewing prednisolone as a dangerous drug and of minimising patient exposure. The same considerations apply to aseptic necrosis of the heads of the long bones.

An intensely painful and quite definite polyarthritis is part of the steroid withdrawal syndrome. At a certain level of dose reduction, often when the dose has been reduced to somewhere between 5 and 10 mg, the patient may develop vomiting and associated electrolyte imbalance, severe disturbance of pattern and quality of sleep, lassitude, malaise and polyarthritis and may indeed become dangerously ill. This is distinct from the picture of recrudescence of the disease for which the patient was being treated with corticosteroids and usually requires a temporary increase in dose of steroid, attention to fluid balance and sometimes even hospital admission.

Thyroid Disease

Musculoskeletal complaints frequently complicate thyroid disease and are often the reason why the patient first requests medical help. Myopathy may complicate both hypothyroidism and hyperthyroidism and may include myasthenic features in the latter. Non-specific aches and pains are almost an integral part of hypothyroidism, and hyperuricaemia (but only very rarely gout) may occur. There is a high incidence of chondrocalcinosis and CPPD in hypothyroidism. Thickening of the soft tissues and of the tendon sheaths is an integral part of myxoedema, and carpal tunnel syndrome is often the presenting complaint. It is important to remember that a more generalised neuropathy may occur in myxoedema and that this will remit completely provided that adequate replacement is prescribed sufficiently early. Cerebellar ataxia may occur due to hypothyroidism. There is an association between hypothyroidism and rheumatoid arthritis. Prominent myopathic involvement in hypothyroidism is called Hoffman's syndrome. Cretinism produces delay in maturation of the epiphyses with irregular ossification and again early diagnosis is all important. In older persons hypothyroidism is frequently due to autoimmune thyroid disease, which in turn may be associated with Sjögren's syndrome and the other organ-specific autoimmune diseases. A lupus-like syndrome may be associated both with hypothyroidism and with Graves' disease, which in turn may be complicated by exophthalmos, pretibial myxoedema and thyroid acropachy. These last manifestations are caused by antireceptor antibody.

Pituitary Disease

Hyperuricaemia may be associated with congenital vasopressin-resistant diabetes insipidus and gout may occur. Since diuretics are often used in this condition, recognition of hyperuricaemia may be important. Acromegaly may be associated with polyostotic fibrous dysplasia which involves the small bones of the hands and feet as well as the vertebral bodies, and this condition may also occur in hypothyroidism and Cushing's syndrome. Apart from these features, the musculoskeletal manifestations of acromegaly are of considerable interest, and as the endocrinologist becomes better able to cope with the primary problem so more and more of these patients survive to develop arthropathies. Early in the disease there is overgrowth of all connective elements, including even cartilage, giving the lie to the idea that chondrocytes are inert. Thereafter the patient develops what looks like a florid form of osteoarthritis. Radiological features are distinctive and include "tufting" of the terminal phalanges, increase in joint space and exuberant osteophytosis. Chondrocalcinosis is common, as is CPPD. In the axial skeleton there is widening of the disc spaces and osteophytosis and the bony proliferation may mimick Forrestier's disease. Clinically the most common presentations are carpal tunnel syndrome, back pain, peripheral joint pain and Raynaud's phenomenon.

Hypoparathyroidism and Hyperparathyroidism

Hypoparathyroidism may be associated with a characteristic shortening of the fourth and fifth metacarpals seen clinically as a deformed hand with skin "dimpling", and with slipped femoral epiphysis. Often the hormone deficiency leads to widespread ectopic soft tissue calcification and in the spine the appearance may mimic Forrestier's disease. Rarely hyperuricaemia due to a renal tubular mechanism may complicate postoperative hypoparathyroidism.

In patients with hyperparathyroidism, hyperuricaemia may occur but the mechanism of this is not known. Gout has been described but it is conceivable that at least some of these patients may instead have been suffering from CPPD, and there is no doubt about the increased frequency of both calcinosis and CPPD in hyperparathyroidism. Indeed, the link between these two conditions may be even more important than has been suspected previously. A proportion of patients with CPPD have been shown to have previously unsuspected elevations of serum parathormone. The relationship between the endocrinopathies, disturbances of iron metabolism and of magnesium and CPPD are in a fascinating state of flux at the moment.

Patients with hyperparathyroidism may develop a peripheral polyarthritis which closely resembles rheumatoid arthritis with synovial proliferation and juxta-articular erosions. The primary lesion, however, appears to be in subchondral bone and certainly there are often conspicuous cystic changes in bone. Additional manifestations include widespread ectopic calcification and a syndrome of acute pericapsulitis which may be caused by calcium hydroxyapatite. This may also affect the entheses and tendon rupture may occur.

Sarcoidosis

Arthritis is a major manifestation of sarcoidosis and may be the presenting feature. There are two quite distinct sarcoid arthritis syndromes. In the first the patient presents acutely with an acute, effusive, non-destructive, inflammatory, symmetrical polyarthritis which is often associated with hilar adenopathy and erythema nodosum. The prognosis is excellent and the patient should be managed with reassurance and a single NSAID such as indomethacin. This is most common in young adults.

However, sarcoidosis may also present as a chronic destructive often asymmetrical lesion of the bone or joint and the prognosis then must be more guarded. This presentation is most common in Negroes in hot countries and there are usually clinical and laboratory features of involvement elsewhere, e.g. chronic uveitis, skin lesions or disease in the lung or liver. Eosinophilia, hypercalcaemia, hyperimmunoglobulinaemia and hyperuricaemia may be found. Tests for the presence of circulating rheumatoid factor may be positive and the tuberculin test negative. This may be a conspicuously destructive disease and all of the non-specific methods of management may be required.

Hypertrophic Osteoarthropathy

Hypertrophic osteoarthropathy is a chronic periostitis of the distal ends of the long bones of the extremities presenting with bilateral symmetrical painful swelling of the wrists and ankles. It is usually associated with finger clubbing and may be accompanied by a chronic effusive non-destructive synovitis. Management of the local problem is usually simple, the important thing being to make the diagnosis and then to search for the associated more ominous disease.

Respiratory Tract

There are several interactions between arthritis and the respiratory system, ranging from the relationship between bronchiectasis or *Mycoplasma pneumoniae* infection and rheumatoid arthritis to involvement of the pleura or lung substance in the multisystem diseases.

Gastrointestinal and Hepatic Disorders

The musculoskeletal system is closely associated, often bidirectionally, with disorders of these organs. The most obvious connection centres upon iatrogenesis, the most common side-effects of the NSAID drugs being gastrointestinal in nature (Chap. 14). The intimate involvement of the granulomatous bowel diseases with the seronegative spondarthritides is covered in full in Chap. 10. The association between autoimmune liver disease and the multisystem connective tissue diseases is covered in Chap. 12.

Conclusion

Musculoskeletal manifestations are an integral part of the clinical presentation of many visceral diseases and an important part of the picture of others. When they form the presenting feature of a disease then their recognition may permit the initiation of effective treatment at an earlier stage than might otherwise have been possible. Management in most instances represents a combination of treatment of the underlying disease together with particular attention to local treatment of the affected joint.

Further Reading

Altman RD, Tenenbaum J (1981) Hypertrophic osteoarthropathy. In: Kelly W, Harris ED Jr, Ruddy S, Sledge CB (1981) Textbook of rheumatology, 1st edn. Saunders, Philadelphia London Toronto, Chap 103

Aron DC, Tyrell JB, Fitzgerald PA, Findling JW, Forsham PH (1981) Cushing's syndrome; problems in diagnosis. Medicine 60: 28–35

Bluestone R (1981) Arthropathies associated with endocrine disorders. In: Kelly W, Harris ED Jr, Ruddy S, Sledge CB (1981) Textbook of rheumatology, 1st edn. Saunders, Philadelphia London Toronto, Chap 101

Bole GG (1981) Arthritis associated with hyperlipidaemia and hypercholesterolaemia. In: Kelly W, Harris ED Jr, Ruddy S, Sledge CB (1981) Textbook of rheumatology, 1st edn. Saunders, Philadelphia London Toronto, Chap 102

Bramble MC, Blake DR, White T, Sly J, Kerr DNS (1980) Ionised calcium in rheumatoid arthritis; effect of NSAID Br Med J 281: 841–844

Caldwell DS (1981) Musculoskeletal syndromes associated with malignancy. In: Kelly W, Harris ED Jr, Ruddy S, Sledge CB (eds) Textbook of rheumatology, 1st edn. Saunders, Philadelphia London Toronto, Chap 104

Clarke AK, Galbraith RM, Hamilton EB, Williams R (1978) Rheumatic disorders in primary biliary cirrhosis. Ann Rheum Dis 37: 42–47

Cox DW, Huber O (1976) Rheumatoid arthritis and alpha-1 antitrypsin. Lancet I: 1216–1217

Geddes DM, Corrin B, Brewerton DA, Davies RT, Turner-Warwick M (1978) Progressive airways obliteration in adults and its association with rheumatoid disease. J Med 46: 427–444

Grennan DM, Howie AD, Moran F, Buchanan WW (1978) Pulmonary involvement in S.L.E. Ann Rheum Dis 37: 536–539

Hamilton EBD (1975) Arthritis of hyperparathyroidism, haemachromatosis and Wilson's disease. Saunders, Philadelphia London Toronto (Clin Rheum Dis, vol 1, pp 109–123)

Kennedy AC, Allen BF, Rooney PJ (1979) Hypercalcaemia in rheumatoid arthritis; an investigation of its causes and implications. Ann Rheum Dis 38: 401–412

Mainardi CL, Levine PH (1981) Haemophilia and arthritis. In: Kelly W, Harris ED Jr, Ruddy S, Sledge CB (1981) Textbook of rheumatology, 1st edn. Saunders, Philadelphia London Toronto, Chap 99

Maury CPJ, Teppo A (1982) Mechanism of reduced amyloid A degrading activity in the serum of patients with secondary amyloidosis. Lancet II: 234–237

Mills PR, Sturrock RD (1982) Clinical associations between arthritis and liver disease. Ann Rheum Dis 41: 295–307

Pastan RS, Cohen AS (1978) The rheumatological manifestations of diabetes mellitus. Med Clin North Am 62: 829–839

Rooney PJ, Ballantyne D, Buchanan WW (1975) Disorders of the locomotor system associated with abnormalities of lipid metabolism and the lipoidoses. Saunders, Philadelphia London Toronto Clin Rheum Dis, vol 1, pp 163–193

Schumacher HR (1981) Arthritis associated with sickle cell disease and other haemaglobinopathies. In: Kelly W, Harris ED Jr, Ruddy S, Sledge CB (eds) Textbook of rheumatology, 1st edn. Saunders, Philadelphia London Toronto, Chap 100

Taylor R, Clarke F, Griffiths IDG, Weeke J (1980) Prospective study of the effect of fenclofenac on thyroid function tests. Br Med J 281: 911–912

Wright JR, Calkins E (1980) Clinical-pathological differentiation of common amyloid syndromes. Medicine 60: 429–448

8 Rheumatoid Disease and Management of Extra-articular Features

Introduction

There is now sufficient clinical, epidemiological, pharmacological and immunogenetic evidence to demonstrate that rheumatoid arthritis is not a single disease. Rather the term describes a syndrome comprising a non-specific progressive chronic inflammatory symmetrical peripheral polyarthritis, seropositivity for serum IgM rheumatoid factor and juxta-articular erosive changes on joint X-ray (Table 8.1).

Table 8.1. Definition of rheumatoid arthritis[a]

1. Inflammatory symmetrical peripheral polyarthritis
2. Seropositivity for IgM rheumatoid factor[b]
3. Juxta-articular erosions on X-ray

[a] These three criteria interrelate in the nature of overlapping Venn functions. Thus each may exist on its own, in association with one of the other two or in association with both of the other two; only the latter condition provides a secure basis for the diagnosis of classical rheumatoid arthritis.
[b] Depends upon local laboratory but test selected must fulfil sensitivity and specificity criteria (1:32 for the Waaler-Rose test)

The American Rheumatism Association criteria for the diagnosis of rheumatoid arthritis, which are under seige at present and will require revision in the near future, are as follows (Ropes et al. 1958):

1. Morning stiffness
2. Pain on motion or tenderness of at least one joint (observed by a physician)
3. Swelling (soft tissue thickening or fluid—not bony overgrowth alone) of at least one joint observed by a physician
4. Swelling (observed by a physician) of at least one other joint (any interval

free of joint symptoms between the two joint involvements may not be more than 3 months)

5. Symmetrical joint swelling (observed by a physician) with simultaneous involvement of the same joint on both sides of the body (bilateral involvement of PIP, MCP or MTP joints is acceptable without absolute symmetry). DIP joint involvement alone will not satisfy this criterion

6. Subcutaneous nodules (observed by a physician) over bony prominences, on extensor surfaces or in juxta-articular regions

7. X-ray changes typical of rheumatoid arthritis (which must include bony decalcification localised to or greatest around the involved joints and not just degenerative changes)

8. Positive agglutination test

9. Poor mucin precipitate from synovial fluid

10. Characteristic changes in synovial membrane with three or more of the following: marked villous hypertrophy, proliferation of superficial synovial cells often with palisading, marked infiltration of chronic inflammatory cells with a tendency to form lymphoid nodules, deposition of compact fibrin either on the surface or interstitially and foci of cell necrosis.

11. Characteristic histological changes in nodules showing granulomatous foci with central zones of cell necrosis surrounded by proliferating fixed cells, peripheral fibrosis and chronic, often perivascular, inflammatory cell infiltrate.

In criteria 1—5 the joint signs must be continuous for at least 6 weeks. *Classical rheumatoid arthritis* is diagnosed when seven of the above criteria are present, *definite rheumatoid arthritis* with five, and *probable rheumatoid arthritis* with three. The diagnosis of *possible rheumatoid arthritis* requires two of the following criteria and the total duration of joint symptoms must be at least 3 weeks:

1. Morning stiffness
2. Tenderness or pain on motion
3. History or observation of joint swelling
4. Subcutaneous nodules
5. Raised ESR or CRP
6. Scleritis (this is now recognised to be in error—editor's note)

Note: Any one of a list of 20 exclusions (Currey 1978) invalidates the diagnosis.

The clinical features and the non-articular complications which may be encountered in this syndrome are summarised in Table 8.2.

The syndrome afflicts large numbers of people (one and a half million in the United Kingdom) in most of the developed countries throughout the world. There are variations in prevalence both geographically and ethnically. It is more common and more severe in temperate climates and the vasculitic complications in particular are much less common in the tropics. Urban blacks are affected more commonly and more severely than rural blacks from the same ethnic origin in South Africa. In the United Kingdom rheumatoid arthritis is responsible for a considerable amount of time lost from work and for a large proportion of general practitioners' time. Afflicting as it does young adults at the peak of their wage-earning potential or in the case of young females when they are most involved in raising their families, it tends to exert a disproportionately large impact upon the community in financial terms. There is some evidence to suggest that this syndrome was rare in Britain until the

Table 8.2. Extra-articular features of rheumatoid disease

Haematological	Normochromic normocytic anaemia "of chronic disease"
	Hypochromic microcytic iron deficiency anaemia (often iatrogenic)
	Aplastic anaemia (often iatrogenic)
	    Any variety and combination of types of anaemia may occur
	    Depression of one or all of the formed elements likewise may occur
	    The association of leucopenia, splenomegaly, recurrent leg
	        ulceration and often inactive destructive longstanding
	        rheumatoid arthritis is termed "Felty's syndrome"

Subcutaneous nodules	
Vasculitis	

Periperal neuropathy	Mononeuritis multiplex
	Symmetrical peripheral sensorimotor neuropathy
	    (The more prominent the motor component, the worse the
	        prognosis)

Gastrointestinal	Dyspepsia, often iatrogenic
	Gastrointestinal blood loss—both regular small volume loss and rarely
	    acute haemorrhage may occur
	The GI tract may also be involved in vasculitis or amyloidosis
	A high proportion of patients have abnormalities in liver function
	    tests, especially rises in liver enzymes. A much smaller proportion
	    have immunological and fewer still pathological evidence of
	    autoimmune liver diseases such as positive mitochondrial antibody
	    and primary biliary cirrhosis or positive smooth muscle antibody
	    and active chronic hepatitis.

Pulmonary	Pleurisy with or without effusion Caplan's syndrome Fibrosing alveolitis Non-pneumoconiotic pulmonary nodules Pulmonary arterial disease
Cardiac	Pericarditis Valvulitis, especially aortic and mitral Vasculitis Granulomatous infiltration of the myocardium
Ocular	Episcleritis Scleritis, scleromalacia perforans Ocular features of the sicca syndrome
Lymphadenopathy	Almost one-third of patients have lymph node enlargement, a smaller proportion having a palpable spleen
Renal	Despite the present worries, the evidence is against the proposal that rheumatoid disease produces a major impact upon the kidney
Other systemic features	Muscle, skin and nail lesions may be produced by the effects of the disease or its treatment and are referred to elsewhere in this text

nineteenth century, that it has reached a peak in the middle part of the present century and that successive generations are presenting less frequently and with less severe disease.

Although presentation may occur in a variety of ways, ranging from carpal tunnel syndrome, monoarthritis or a febrile wasting illness to an isolated extra-articular manifestation, the fully expressed disease is nevertheless remarkably uniform in its characteristics.

In the hand the distribution is so distinctive that the diagnosis can often be made on this basis alone. The distribution of involvement is different from both osteoarthritis and the inflammatory arthritides such as JCP (juvenile chronic polyarthritis) or psoriatic arthritis. The peripheral distribution contrasts with the seronegative spondarthritides such as ankylosing spondylitis and the symmetry of involvement differs from the metabolic arthritides such as gout.

The evolution of the disease is marked by wide fluctuations in disease activity which may occur surprisingly quickly. These patients may change quite considerably even within 1 week and there is a noticeable diurnal variability. Such changes in disease activity are unsettling for the patient and frustrate the considerable efforts which have been made in the field of assessment of proposed new antirheumatic drugs. Patients should have the course of their disease plotted as accurately as possible, this being an important part of decision making in therapeutics (see Fig. 1.2). It is also interesting and important to attempt to determine whether or not within the individual there are features which may affect disease activity predictably. Whereas it is well known that pregnancy or the development of severe jaundice may induce remission, it is less often emphasised that bereavement, redundancy, intercurrent illness or accident and depression may precipitate an exacerbation.

The course of the disease is complicated by a trend underlying that of disease activity, which may best be described as irreversible destruction. This may behave quite differently from the measures which reflect disease activity such as pain and tenderness indices, the duration and severity of morning stiffness and the laboratory indices of acute phase protein involvement such as ESR or CRP (C-reactive protein) and is best expressed in terms of functional index or X-ray stage. The determination of grip strength is a composite index which may include variable proportions of each of these separable processes. This graph of underlying destructive disease should be plotted separately from the graph of disease activity and presents different therapeutic goals. The tendency is for this graph to describe an early phase of deterioration followed by many years of plateau, and in the last phase of the disease it is common to note underlying improvement rather than deterioration; thus the individual prognosis must take account of the pattern of disease throughout its course and the stage at which one is seeing the patient.

A sequence of events can be discerned in any single peripheral joint. The single cell layer of superficial type A (macrophage-like phagocytic cell replete with endocytic lysosomal vesicles) and type B (synthetic cells with abundant endoplasmic reticulum) synoviocytes proliferates and is thrown into folds and villi. The subsynovial cells, including the endothelial vascular cells, also proliferate and in addition there is a dense infiltrate of monocytic cells from the circulation. In the synovial fluid, which is increased in amount and is abnormal in constitution, polymorphonuclear cells predominate, but in the subsynovium macrophages and lymphocytes are the cells most frequently seen. The B-lymphocyte lineage is actively involved in the synthesis of IgG and IgM rheumatoid factors. However, many of the lymphocytes in rheumatoid synovium are T cells and it is likely that the OKT4 marked "helper" cell subset is overrepresented compared with the OKT8 cytotoxic or suppressor T cell. Recent evidence suggests that an as yet uncharacterised antigen presenting cell, analogous to the Langerhans' cell of skin, is present in rheumatoid synovium. Certainly it is now obvious that the synovium in this condition becomes a highly active immunological organ of the first importance.

Pathophysiologically there is increased perfusion of this highly cellular tissue, but the increase is not sufficient to meet the demands of the tissue and there is a reduction in the local pH and an increase in local lactate concentration. The membrane is abnormally permeable to large molecular weight proteins and the viscoelastic properties of normal synovial fluid are lost. The synovial fluid contains an abundance of abnormal constituents, including immune complexes, acute phase proteins, neutral and acidic proteolytic enzymes (although these are present in inhibitor excess) and abnormal proteoglycans. In addition the glucose concentration is reduced.

There is evidence of an abnormal metabolic and hormonal balance in patients with rheumatoid arthritis. Hepatocyte involvement is marked by the acute phase protein response with elevation of CRP, haptoglobin, kininogen, α-2-macroglobulin and α-2-antitrypsin and a reduction in serum albumin. These changes are accompanied by a reduction in serum zinc and an increase in serum copper. It is likely that these events are all linked. As serum zinc falls, a factor (?interleukin 1) is released from polymorphonuclear leucocytes which stimulates the hepatocyte to increase its uptake of the essential precursor amino acids such as histidine, the concentration of which then falls in serum. These precursors are then used as the building blocks for the acute phase proteins such as caeruloplasmin, and the resultant rise in its concentration produces the increase in serum copper. Other evidence of liver involvement in this disease includes the frequent presence of hepatomegaly or hepatosplenomegaly, increases in alkaline phosphatase and other "liver" enzymes and the presence in some patients of either chronic active hepatitis with a smooth muscle autoantibody or primary biliary cirrhosis with antimitochondrial autoantibody. It has been suggested that there are profound disturbances in calcium metabolism, but whether or not this is related to drug therapy has not yet been elucidated. Likewise, serum radioimmunoreactive gastrin may be elevated but the mechanism of this is obscure. In addition, pulmonary, cardiac, neurological, eye, mouth and skin disease may occur and may antedate or be interspersed during the course of articular manifestations (Tables 8.2, 8.3).

Thus rheumatoid arthritis should be called rheumatoid disease. There is evidence of widespread involvement of many organs and tissues and of a profound metabolic disturbance.

Many of the later chapters of this text are focussed upon the management of the articular component of the disease (Chaps. 13–18) and therefore the remainder of this chapter is devoted to the management of the extra-articular features.

Management of Systemic Disease

Failure to recognise rheumatoid arthritis as a systemic disease with many extra-articular manifestations is common. The extent of involvement varies greatly and does not necessarily parallel the severity of, or variation in, joint symptoms.

The Eye

Expert ophthalmological assistance in monitoring and managing rheumatoid patients is indispensible. Properly treated morbidity from eye involvement can be minimised.

Keratoconjunctivitis sicca (Sjögren's syndrome, Tables 8.3, 8.4) is best managed by frequent instillation of hydroxymethyl cellulose eye drops. Most patients derive considerable symptomatic benefit and, given understanding of the rationale of the treatment, will persevere with therapy as prescribed; attention needs to be paid, however, to the actual instillation of drops in patients who have poor hand function and require assistance. Occasionally inspissated mucus may necessitate the use of a mucolytic agent and in rare instances coagulation of the nasolacrimal duct is indicated. The dry eye is susceptible to infection which requires prompt identification and treatment.

Episcleritis is relatively benign and does not usually require treatment. Recurrences are common, however, and occasionally a topical steroid is indicated.

Scleritis, though much less common, is potentially much more serious, and careful monitoring during treatment with a topical steroid such as betamethasone sodium phosphate 0.1% eye drops or ointment is essential. In severe scleritis systemic steroid may be tried but may fail to control the inflammation. In these cases cytotoxic drugs have been used, but without documented evidence of efficacy.

Glaucoma or *cataract* may complicate rheumatoid eye disease or steroid treatment and this possibility must be borne in mind so that appropriate therapy can be instituted.

The Mouth

Xerostomia is difficult to treat effectively. Segments of an orange or other citrus fruit sucked intermittently through the day and night or simple mouth washes are

Table 8.3. Sjögren's syndrome[a]

Feature	Diagnostic/assessment tests
Dry eyes (keratoconjunctivitis sicca)	History/clinical examination Rose Bengal staining Schirmer tear test Slit lamp examination of eye
Dry mouth (xerostomia)	History/clinical examination Salivary flow rate Sialography Salivary scintiscanning Minor salivary gland biopsy
Any multisystem connective tissue disorder	In the majority of patients rheumatoid arthritis is the CT disease but in others it may be SLE, PSS, dermatomyositis or even autoimmune liver disease

[a] "Sjögren's syndrome" = any two or more of the above three features
Keratoconjunctivitis sicca and xerostomia alone = "sicca complex"
In recent terminology "primary" Sjögren's syndrome = keratoconjunctivitis sicca, while "secondary" Sjögren's syndrome = either or both of these together with an associated connective tissue disease

Table 8.4. Extraocular and extraoral clinical features of Sjögren's syndrome

Respiratory tract	Dryness of the upper respiratory tract and associated structures, including the external auditory meatus, causing secondary infection or conduction deafness
Mouth and throat	Periodontal disease and rampant dental caries Dysphagia Postcricoid web/Plummer-Vinson syndrome
Skin	Dryness, chronic inflammation of the sweat glands Hyperglobulinaemic purpura Raynaud's phenomenon
Vagina	Dyspareunia/secondary infection
Gastrointestinal	Chronic atrophic gastritis/achlorhydria/pernicious anaemia Primary biliary cirrhosis Chronic active hepatitis Chronic pancreatitis
Thyroid	Hashimoto's thyroiditis Primary hypothyroidism
Kidney	Renal tubular acidosis Loss of concentrating ability, aminoaciduria, glycosuria
Central nervous system	Cranial nerve lesions Peripheral neuropathy
Reticuloendothelial	Lymphadenopathy and splenomegaly
Drug allergy (especially penicillin)	
Neoplasia	Extra- and intrasalivary lymphoreticular neoplasms (especially in those who have undergone irradiation), malignant lymphomas, Waldenström's macroglobulinaemia, Franklin's heavy chain disease
Haematological	In the sicca syndrome alone the haemoglobin is often surprisingly normal. However, a Coomb's positive haemolytic anaemia may occur. Leucopenia, lymphopenia and thrombocytopenia are common

of some symptomatic benefit. Meticulous attention to dental hygiene will help protect the patient from caries, which occur more commonly in xerostomia, and prompt treatment of complications such as oral candida or salivary gland infection is required.

Nodules

Second line drugs may reduce the size and number of nodules but in the absence of appropriate articular indications they should not be prescribed for this reason alone. Cosmetic removal is not recommended since the nodules recur and poor wound healing is common. The most important therapy for nodules (especially those occurring over the sacrum) is a simple mechanical one; namely to protect them from trauma wherever possible. If they break down and become infected, antibiotic cover and devoted nursing will be necessary.

Pulmonary Disease

There is no proven effective therapy for rheumatoid lung disease. Exclusion of alternative causes for pleural effusions and pulmonary nodules, e.g. neoplasm or tuberculosis, is vital. Prompt vigorous management of pulmonary infections which are more common in the rheumatoid patient, proscription of cigarette smoking and in coal miners referral to the pneumoconiosis board are the only positive contributions which the clinician can make. Fortunately, uncomplicated rheumatoid lung disease rarely leads to significant respiratory impairment. If possible, aside from diagnostic indications, it is generally best to leave alone the small or moderate sized effusions which are the most common complication of rheumatoid arthritis in the chest. The patient with rapidly advancing small airways disease has a very poor prognosis but fortunately this is most unusual.

Cardiac Disease

Effective treatment for cardiac involvement in rheumatoid arthritis has not been established. Pericarditis is often intermittent and may be managed by simple anti-inflammatory drugs and analgesics. In the rare event of cardiac tamponade, heroic doses of steroid have been used without firm evidence of efficacy. Pericardiectomy is occasionally required. Conduction defects are seldom seen, and proof of vasculitis as a cause of myocardial infarction is well nigh impossible to obtain ante mortem.

The development of aortic or mitral incompetence is rare but may lead to cardiac decompensation and require conventional anti-failure measures. Early liaison with cardiologist colleagues will allow appropriate timing of valve surgery, should this become necessary.

Neuropathy

The first step in management is precise diagnosis and exclusion of all treatable causes, in particular in this instance iatrogenesis. The second line drugs, e.g. gold, are possibly implicated in this respect and other drugs, e.g. indomethacin, may be responsible. It is vitally important to exclude entrapment, whether peripherally or near the cord, as a possible cause of neurological symptoms and signs. Once this has been accomplished an expectant non-interventionist policy is best. Only in the presence of clearly advancing signs should escalation to more powerful drug therapy or neurosurgery be considered.

Depression (Table 8.5)

Although many patients with rheumatoid arthritis or any other chronic destructive inflammatory joint disease become depressed at some stage in their disease, few will benefit from antidepressant drugs or ECT. A depressive reaction to a painful chronic disease and loss of independence should be managed by mobilising every possible resource to minimise pain and disability. It is, however, important to differentiate this reaction from coincidental depression occurring in an arthritic patient. While the distinction may at times be difficult, psychiatric counselling and antidepressant medication may be needed in the latter group. Coincidental depression is marked both by positive clinical features such as a positive family history, fluctuations divorced from those of the inflammatory joint disease, and perhaps other features of a unipolar lithium-responsive endogenous depression such as delusions or early morning waking as well as negative clinical clues.

Table 8.5. Depression in chronic inflammatory joint disease

Coincidental depression	Varies independently of arthritis
	Often antedates the arthritis
	Positive features, e.g. unipolar, lithium responsive, positive family history, early a.m. waking, delusions, retardation
	Treat along conventional lines
Iatrogenic	Onset related to medication
	Withdraw offending drug
Integral part of disease	Severity fluctuates in proportion to measures of constitutional disease activity, e.g. pain and tenderness indices, ESR, Hb, serum albumin, APP
Related to functional impairment (="frustration")	Severity proportional to X-ray stage, functional index etc. Treat with functional aids or reconstructive surgery
"Reactive" depression— antidepressant drugs	Decide on the therapeutic goal
	Institute single antidepressant, N.B. adequate dose, adequate time! Monitor to the attainment of the therapeutic goal or withdraw

It is most important to exclude iatrogenesis when withholding the offending agent may be all that is required. Corticosteroids are notorious in this respect, as is indomethacin, but any of the NSAID group of drugs may be responsible.

Amyloidosis

No treatment has been shown to produce unequivocal benefit in amyloidosis secondary to rheumatoid arthritis. Penicillamine, cytotoxics, dimethylsulphoxide and colchicine have been suggested, but a definitive study has yet to be performed. If joint disease activity warrants penicillamine or cytotoxic drugs, these should be continued despite the problems of monitoring penicillamine in the face of heavy proteinuria.

Management of the patient with amyloid centres mainly on general measures suitable for the degree of renal impairment or, in the case of malabsorption, elimination of complicating bacterial overgrowth.

Rupture of a Peripheral Joint Cavity

Rupture of a peripheral joint cavity is a common event in the course of rheumatoid arthritis and is very often misdiagnosed. This topic is covered more fully in Chap. 2.

Presentation with Marked Constitutional Features

Weight loss, anaemia, lymphadenopathy or leucopenia may be the major problems at one or other stage in the evolution of the disease and it must be borne in mind that rheumatoid arthritis is a wasting disease. Frequently the attending clinician is faced with the vexing question of whether or not such features may safely be ascribed to the primary disease, i.e. rheumatoid arthritis, or whether some other process such as malignancy or infection has supervened. Too often no help can be given to that clinician and the only recourse is to rely upon clinical judgement. Laboratory tests presently available in such a circumstance are frequently unhelpful. One is then left to judge clinically whether or not the degree of, or the rate of development of, weight loss, anaemia or lymphadenopathy is in proportion to the activity of the primary disease. One rough rule is that any node which is disproportionately enlarged and any node above the clavicle should be biopsied. Again, the compilation of accurate ongoing graphs of progression may be of assistance. It may become obvious that the change in haemoglobin concentration over the preceding period is distinctly different from the state of the arthritis during that same period, drawing attention to the possibility of drug-induced gastrointestinal haemorrhage, or some other cause of anaemia.

Articular Presentations of Unusual Significance

Although this section is devoted to non-articular problems there are two circumstances of particular moment which should be covered in this context:

1. Complications occasioned by disease in the atlantoaxial region and in the cervical spine may be life threatening. The florid case with overt neurological symptoms and signs needs little emphasis except to call it to mind. However, the presentation will often be less clamant, the patient merely going "off her feet", and this demands a higher index of suspicion. Any sudden change in an otherwise stable patient must be investigated thoroughly, and it is good practice to occasionally X-ray the cervical spine as a routine measure in any patient with severe disease. In addition meticulous neurological examination is mandatory.

2. In a similar vein, the only way to avoid missing supervening infection within the joint of a patient with chronic rheumatoid arthritis is again to have a high index of suspicion and to look askance at any individual joint and any patient where there is sudden deterioration. This is a particular risk in patients who have undergone reconstructive surgery.

Further Reading

Aaseth J, Munthe E, Forre O, Steinnes E (1978) Trace elements in the serum and urine of patients wth rheumatoid arthritis. Scand J Rheumatol 7: 237–240

Alspaugh MA, Whaley K (1981) Sjögren's syndrome. In: Kelly W, Harris ED Jr, Ruddy S, Sledge CB (eds) Textbook of rheumatology, 1st edn. Saunders, Philadelphia London Toronto, Chap 62

Anderson LG, Talal N (1971) The spectrum of benign to malignant lymphoproliferation in Sjögren's syndrome. Clin Exp Immunol 9: 199–221

Buchanan WW (1978) Clinical features of rheumatoid arthritis. In: Scott JT (ed) Copeman's textbook of the rheumatic diseases, 5th edn. Churchill Livingstone, Edinburgh London New York, Chap. 13

Carson DA (1981) Rheumatoid factor. In: Kelly W, Harris ED Jr, Ruddy S, Sledge CB (eds) Textbook of rheumatology, 1st edn. Saunders, Philadelphia London Toronto, Chap 44

Cooper NS, Soren A, McEwan C, Rosenberger JL (1981) Diagnostic specificity of synovial lesions. Hum Pathol 12: 314–328

Currey HLF (1978) Aetiology and pathogenesis of rheumatoid arthritis. In: Scott JT (ed) Copeman's textbook of the rheumatic diseases, 5th edn. Churchill Livingstone, Edinburgh London New York, Chap. 11

Denman AM (1978) Rheumatoid arthritis—a virus disease? J Clin Pathol 31 [Suppl 12]: 132–143

Dewar PJ (in press) HLA antigens. In: Dick WC, Moll JMH (eds) Recent advances in rheumatology, 3rd edn. Churchill Livingstone, Edinburgh London New York

Duthie JJR (1964) Course and prognosis in rheumatoid arthritis. Ann Rheum Dis 23: 193–204

Grennan DM, Anderson JA, Kennedy AC, Mitchell WS, Dick WC, Buchanan WW (1975) Relationship between haemoglobin and other clinical and laboratory parameters in rheumatoid arthritis. Curr Med Res Opin 3(2): 104–108

Harris ED Jr (1981) Rheumatoid arthritis; the clinical spectrum. In: Kelly W, Harris ED Jr, Ruddy S, Sledge CB (eds) Textbook of rheumatology, 1st edn. Saunders, Philadelphia London Toronto, Chap 60

Janossy G, Duke O, Poulter LW, Panayi G, Bofill M, Goldstein G (1981) Rheumatoid arthritis; a disease of T-lymphocyte/macrophage immunoregulation. Lancet II: 839–842

Johnson PM (1979) Stimuli for anti-IgG antibody production in rheumatoid arthritis. In: Panayi GS, Johnson PM (eds) Immunopathogenesis of rheumatoid arthritis. Reedbooks, Surrey, pp 45–50

Kennedy AC, Allam BF, Boyle IT, Nuki G, Rooney PJ, Buchanan WW (1975) Abnormalities in mineral metabolism suggestive of parathyroid overactivity in rheumatoid arthritis. Curr Med Res Opin 3(6): 345–358

McGavin DDM, Williamson J, Forrestier JV, Foulds WS, Buchanan WW, Dick WC, Lee P, MacSween RNM, Whaley K (1976) Episcleritis and scleritis. Br J Ophthalmol 60: 192–224

Malcolm AJ (in press) Diagnostic pathology in rheumatology. In: Dick WC, Moll JMH (eds) Recent advances in rheumatology, 3rd edn. Churchill Livingstone, Edinburgh London New York

Mills PR, MacSween RNM, Dick WC, More IA, Watkinson G (1980) Liver disease in rheumatoid arthritis. Scott Med J 25: 18–22

Mowat AG, Hothersall TE, Aitchison WRC (1969) Nature of anaemia in rheumatoid arthritis. Ann Rheum Dis 28: 303–309

Pattison E, Prothero K, Pringle RM, Kennedy AC, Dick WC (1973) Reduction in haemoglobin after knee joint surgery. Ann Rheum Dis 32: 582

Queiros MV, Sancho MRH, Caetano JM (1982) HLA Dr4 antigen and IgM rheumatoid factors. J Rheumatol 9: 370–373

Raff HV, Picker LJ, Stobo JD (1980) Macrophage heterogeneity in man. J Exp Med 152: 581–593

Rheinherz EL, Schlossman SF (1981) The characterisation and function of human immunoregulatory T-lymphocyte subsets. Immunol Today 2: 69–74

Rhind VM, Bird HA, Wright V (1980) A comparison of clinical assessments of disease activity in rheumatoid arthritis. Ann Rheum Dis 39: 135–137

Robertson MDJ, Hart FD, White WF, Nuki G, Boardman PL (1968) Rheumatoid lymphadenopathy. Ann Rheum Dis 27: 253–260

Ropes MW, Bennet GA, Cobb S, Jacox R, Jessa RA (1958) Revision of diagnostic criteria for rheumatoid arthritis. Bull Rheum Dis 9: 175–176

Rose NR (1981) Autoimmune diseases. Sci Am (Feb) 70–81

Stastney P (1980) Joint report on rheumatoid arthritis histocompatibility testing. Tissue Antigens 681–686

Whaley K, Webb J (1977) Liver and kidney disease in rheumatoid arthritis. Saunders, Philadelphia London Toronto (Clin Rheum Dis, vol 3, pp 527–547)

Wooley DE, Evanson JM (1980) Present status and future perspectives in collagenase research. In: Woolley DE, Evanson JM (eds) Collagenase in normal and pathological tissue. John Wiley, Chichester, Chap 13.

9 Juvenile Chronic Arthritis

Introduction

This is one of the most exciting areas of medicine at the moment, and recent developments have forced us to change our views in this more than in most other areas. The foundation of these changes in attitude are soundly based on the most reliable long-term data available in rheumatology. At Taplow in England a large group of thoroughly documented children have now been followed up through three generations. This is the epitome of the best of clinical research and serves as a standard for other clinical work in this and in other fields. The eponymous term "Still's disease" should be restricted to patients presenting with a systemic illness, lymphadenopathy, polyserositis, polyarthritis and a distinctive skin rash and should not be used as a ragbag term to conceal the need for thorough clinical documentation. This is said with all respect to George Frederick Still, who himself recognised the heterogeneity of the cases which he described.

Juvenile chronic arthritis (JCA; Table 9.1), also known as juvenile chronic polyarthritis (JCP), is defined as a persistent arthritis afflicting a person of less than 16 years of age. Never has more care been required in the selection of words. Arthritis denotes an inflammatory synovitis, arthralgia being the term employed to indicate pain experienced in the region of a joint in the absence of signs of local inflammation. Tenosynovitis indicates inflammation of the synovium lining tendon sheaths, bursitis being the term used for inflammation within a synovial-lined cavity in soft tissues which may or may not communicate with a joint. Enthesitis describes inflammation at a site of insertion of muscle through ligament or tendon into bone. The word "enthesopathy" indicates pain or dysfunction due to an abnormality at that site without accompanying signs of local inflammation. The basis for most of the problems encountered at the entheses is usually either traumatic or one of the seronegative spondarthritides. The importance of precise description of the site of maximum tenderness has already been stressed (Fig. 1.1).

Table 9.1. Classification of juvenile chronic polyarthritis (ANA, antinuclear factor; RF, rheumatoid factor)

Subgroup	Sex	Age	Joints	Extra-articular features	Laboratory results	Prognosis
Systemic	60% M	Any	Any	Fever, rash Polyserositis Organomegaly (Still's)	ANA−ve RF−ve	25% severe arthritis
RF−ve polyarthritis	90% F	Any	Any	Growth retardation Mild anaemia Slight fever	ANA 25% RF−ve	15% severe arthritis
RF+ve polyarthritis	80% F	Early teens	Any	c.f. adult rheumatoid arthritis	ANA 75% RF+ve	>50% severe arthritis
Pauciarticular with chronic iridocyclitis	80% F	Early childhood	Few (hips)	Few, but 50% have chronic uveitis	ANA 50% RF−ve	Joints good 20% eyes bad
Pauciarticular with sacroiliitis	90% M	Late childhood	Especially hips and sacroiliac joints	Few, but 5%–10% have acute uveitis	ANA−ve RF−ve B27+ve	Many develop ankylosing spondylitis/ other sero−ve spondylitis

Systemic Onset Disease

A proportion (about one-fifth) of children with JCA become systemically ill acutely and present with the constellation of signs and symptoms referred to above. This is equally common in girls and boys and may occur at any age. Indeed, patients presenting apparently for the first time in adult life have been described. Additional evidence separating this syndrome from the other forms of JCA is available in the different HLA haplotype relationships found in these different situations. A conspicuous feature of this type of JCA is the high intermittent fever (103°–105°F) with peaks and even rigors which may be confined to the late afternoon or evening, the temperature falling to normal or even below normal in the interval. Likewise the maculopapular erythematous eruption is evanescent and may be apparent only at the height of the pyrexia. The primary elements are erythematous macules which may show central pallor and are distributed on the trunk and limbs; pruritus is not usually a prominent feature. The eruption may be highlighted by placing the child in a warm bath, and it may be possible to elicit the Koebner phenomenon. The distinctive combination of the rash and the fever together with the other clinical features serve to distinguish this from other diseases which may mimic it, including rheumatic fever, Henoch-Schönlein purpura, osteomyelitis, blood dyscrasias, acute infections of childhood and drug eruptions. The most difficult differential diagnoses at times are from rubella arthritis or in the child with glandular fever (EB virus disease) who develops a skin rash when prescribed ampicillin.

Other extra-articular features also tend to overshadow the arthropathy. Lymphadenopathy may be so pronounced as to suggest lymphoma, and the interpretation of the histological appearance may serve to confuse the uninitiated even further. Hepatomegaly is common and must be distinguished from that produced by drugs such as aspirin or even complicating amyloidosis. Polyserositis is common and 50% of the patients have pericarditis or pleurisy. Polyserositis is the basis of the acute abdominal pain which may present in a manner that can be confused with appendicitis in systemic lupus, in rheumatic fever or in this condition. (Other "medical" conditions which may present in a similar manner include mesenteric adenitis, porphyria, diabetes mellitus, familial mediterranean fever, tabes, posterior nerve root compression and lead poisoning). Less commonly there may be severe involvement of the myocardium or even valvulitis.

These systemic features may wax and wane with exacerbations which may last from days to several months, but rarely does the disease stay active into adult life. A small proportion of children pursue a most aggressive course and it is these children who are most liable to develop amyloidosis.

Constitutional signs include a normochromic normocytic anaemia, marked polymorphonuclear leucocytosis (50 000–60 000 per mm^3) with a predominance of immature forms, and an elevation of all of the acute phase proteins. Immunoglobulin concentrations may be elevated but serum albumin is often reduced. Tests for the presence of circulating immune complexes and autoantibodies including rheumatoid factor and antinuclear factor are usually negative and there are as yet no clearly defined associations with the gene products of the major histocompatibility complex.

Thus the clinical picture is that of a sick child with a multisystem disease and profound constitutional upset. The musculoskeletal manifestations, though often overshadowed by the other clinical features, are well worth documenting since these may make the diagnosis in a sick child. Most children have evidence of articular involvement on careful clinical examination. Monoarthritis may be the most obvious clinical finding but close examination will usually reveal involvement of other joints and it is particularly important to examine the temperomandibular joint in addition to all the other peripheral diarthrodial joints. More commonly the clinical pattern is one of a symmetrical inflammatory peripheral polyarthritis with swelling (soft tissue plus fluid), tenderness over the articular margins and functional disability, e.g. a limp. Pain is often less conspicuous in children. Tenosynovitis and soft tissue subcutaneous or tendinous nodules must be specifically sought. Such nodules have a histological appearance more akin to the nodules of rheumatic fever than to those of adult rheumatoid arthritis.

Radiological examination in early disease is rarely helpful in excluding other conditions. Soft tissue swelling is detected more efficiently by clinical examination and juxta-articular osteopenia is very non-specific. Juxta-articular erosions and cysts and subluxation are late findings.

The prognosis for these children is better than is conventionally appreciated. Sixty to seventy per cent will reach adult life with only moderate or even mild disability. The two most feared and potentially lethal complications are amyloidosis and supervening sepsis.

Polyarticular Seronegative JCA

This represents quite a distinct subgroup, affecting predominantly females (F:M, 9:1) and tending to begin between the ages of 2 and 5 years. There is a peripheral symmetrical pattern which often includes involvement of the distal interphalangeal joints of the upper and lower limbs, this being unusual in adult onset rheumatoid arthritis. The temporomandibular joints and the joints of the cervical spine are frequently involved and epiphyseal growth disturbance and fibrous or even bony ankylosis may be prominent on X-ray. It is extremely unusual for patients with seropositive adult onset rheumatoid arthritis to develop bony ankylosis. The growth disturbances may leave a permanent record that onset was indeed in childhood and this may be a valuable clinical sign in adults in whom the true diagnosis might otherwise have been missed. Inequalities of digit or limb and malocclusion due to micrognathia should raise the suspicion of this pathogenesis. In passing it is worth pointing out that a significant degree of micrognathia requires that the mandibular epiphysis must have been involved and not simply the temporomandibular joint. Lymphadenopathy and hepatosplenomegaly may be detected but are not prominent, and nodules, uveitis and polyserositis are very rare. Anaemia and leucocytosis, if present, are inconspicuous and constitutional signs are minimal. Tests for the presence of serum IgM rheumatoid factor are negative but a proportion of children may show positive tests for antinuclear factor.

The outlook for these children is excellent, over 80% reaching adulthood with only mild or indeed no residual deformity.

Polyarticular Seropositive JCA

A small proportion of children with JCA (about 10%) have a disease which is the exact counterpart of adult rheumatoid arthritis in all respects, even extending to the layer of the eye involved. Ocular inflammation, when present in a child in whom rheumatoid factor is present in serum, affects the episclera and the sclera in contradistinction to the situation in the child with antinuclear factor, where the layer of the eye affected tends to be the uveal tract. Management of these children follows the guidelines recorded elsewhere in this text with the proviso that it is even more important to concentrate upon prevention, for example, of flexion deformities. An additional factor which assumes importance in children is the need to maximise their educational attainment. If such children can be taken through to higher education then this provides them with the best possible protection in later life and the best possible chance to exert some measure of control over their environment. The prospect of having to earn a living as a manual worker is radically different from the prospect of working as a teacher, lawyer, bank manager, doctor or computer operator.

Pauciarticular JCA

A large proportion of children with JCA (more than 50%) suffer from an arthritis which involves conspicuously few (less than four) joints. Such children may also have other distinctive features, including a family history of one of the members of the seronegative spondarthritides, and it is likely that many in this group are experiencing the onset of one of these diseases. At the moment two distinct subgroups are recognised, namely (a) pauciarticular arthritis with chronic iridocyclitis and (b) pauciarticular arthritis with sacroiliitis.

Pauciarticular Arthritis with Chronic Iridocyclitis

These children present few problems from the point of view of their joints and it is important to avoid being lulled into a false sense of security. There is very little evidence of local or systemic activity and extra-articular features are conspicuous by their absence, with the notable and vitally important exception of ocular involvement. These children develop insidiously a sight-threatening anterior uveitis which may be detected early only by regular examinations employing all of the techniques available to an informed and interested ophthalmologist. This is no circumstance for the "routine review" clinic.

This is most common in the female and the joints most commonly involved are the knees, elbows and ankles, often in an asymmetrical pattern. Hips and sacroiliac joints tend to be spared and there is no evidence of a constitutional reaction. The only clue which may be of value is a positive test for antinuclear factor. As yet there are no documented relationships to any of the HLA antigens and rheumatoid factor is absent.

The eyes of these children must be examined at least four times per year. Clinical signs such as photophobia or redness are late in appearing. The iris and ciliary body bear the brunt of the disease and complications include posterior synechiae, band keratopathy, secondary cataract and visual loss. Management requires the expert assistance of the ophthalmologist but the prognosis for sight is not good.

Pauciarticular Arthritis with Sacroiliitis

Approximately 15% of children with JCA, usually boys, will develop a pattern of involvement which in its later stages is identical to that of ankylosing spondylitis. Antinuclear factor is absent, as too is rheumatoid factor, but there is a relationship to HLA-B27. If these children do develop anterior uveitis, then it is usually an acute non-destructive process which does not threaten vision. The peripheral arthritis affects the lower more often than the upper limb joints and is usually asymmetrical. Hips and sacroiliac joints are often involved and enthesitis is conspicuous. In such children the prevention of flexion deformities is the first priority.

Conclusion

It is obvious that a great deal of attention must be focussed upon children. The onset of many of the arthropathies of adult life may be traced to this age group when the history is taken properly, and the opportunities for early prophylactic and preventitive measures are considerable. The problem facing the general practitioner again is to distinguish the significant from the trivial and this is no easy task. An awareness of the family history may help to raise the index of suspicion.

Further Reading

Ansell BM (1977) Joint manifestations in children with juvenile chronic polyarthritis. Arthritis Rheum 20: 204

Ansell BM, Bywaters EGL (1978) Juvenile chronic polyarthritis. In: Scott JT (ed) Copeman's textbook of the rheumatic diseases. Churchill Livingstone, Edinburgh London New York, Chap 14

Cassidy JT (1981) Juvenile rheumatoid arthritis. In: Kelly W, Harris ED Jr, Ruddy S, Sledge CB (eds) Textbook of rheumatology, 1st edn. Saunders, Philadelphia London Toronto, Chap 80

Schaller JG (1978) The arthritides of childhood. In: Dick WC, Buchanan WW (eds) Recent advances in rheumatology. Churchill Livingstone, Edinburgh London New York, p 89

10 The Seronegative Spondarthritides

Introduction

"Seronegative spondarthritides" is a clumsy expression yet it embodies much that is important in clinical rheumatology. The original concept was developed upon a secure basis of solid long-term clinical documentation, notably in the Leeds unit and in Taplow. At an early stage it was recognised that the term "seronegative rheumatoid arthritis" represented a destructive concept, lumping patients together and forcing them to fit the outdated textbook. The development of rheumatology from that time when this false standard was lowered has been one of unfettered advance.

There is considerable room for expansion upon the present nine members of the group, which are:

1. Uncomplicated ankylosing spondylitis
2. Psoriatic arthritis
3. Reiter's syndrome
4. Ulcerative colitis
5. Crohn's disease
6. Whipple's disease
7. Behçet's syndrome
8. Chronic uveitis
9. "Reactive" arthritis (e.g. to *Yersinnia*, campylobacter)

Their unifying characteristics are:

1. Sheep cell agglutination test negative at 1:32
2. Absence of subcutaneous nodules
3. Inflammatory (often asymmetrical) peripheral polyarthritis
4. Sacroiliitis/spondylitis
5. Clinical overlap within patients and their families

It is important to note that in some of the members of the group, one or a group of infectious agents has been incriminated by more or less powerful evidence ranging from the relationship between the cross-reacting enteropathic Gram-negative bacilli (CREG) and ankylosing spondylitis or Reiter's syndrome on the one hand to Whipple's "bacillus" and disease on the other. It is also clear that not all individuals harbouring these organisms will develop one or indeed any of these diseases. Thus the evidence linking these diseases to individual susceptibility, to the HLA-B27 containing haplotype, assumes greater significance. It should be emphasised that the debate between the one- and the two-gene model is by no means resolved. The one-gene model predicts that development of the disease is intimately linked to the HLA-B27 gene product itself whereas the two-gene model argues for the presence on the same chromosome in close proximity to the HLA-B27 gene of a distinct and separate disease-producing gene. Underlying this debate is the concept of "cross-reactivity", which suggests that the responsible gene product is structurally and stereochemically similar to an exogenous organism which may in other circumstances live in symbiosis with the host but which is not clearly distinguished from "self" under these circumstances. It is suggested that antibodies made to structures on the surface of this organism crossreact with host tissue and evoke a local inflammatory and destructive response. Implicit in much of this theorising is that the site or origin and subsequent penetration of the responsible organism is the gastrointestinal tract. In sexually acquired reactive arthritis (SARA) the important site is presumed to be the urogenital tract.

This debate is not restricted to rheumatology although much of the original data and hypotheses stemmed from that field. The outcome of this debate is important to endocrinology, neurology, gastroenterology and nephrology, and much of the data generated from careful clinicolaboratory studies in diabetes and in families of patients with diabetes is highly relevant. The important debate today is no longer "the seed *or* the soil" but instead concerns the unravelling of the different admixtures of each operating in different bacteriological and clinical milieux. Thus the group of diseases called the seronegative spondarthritides are the focus for some of the most exciting debates in medicine today.

Ankylosing Spondylitis

Ankylosing spondylitis is a disease which primarily affects the axial skeleton, and in particular the sacroiliac joints. The disease in its most florid form is more common in the male but recent evidence suggests that milder forms of the disease are more common in the female than was suspected previously. It is likely that onset is in the early years of life but the disease does not become overt until the second or often even the third decade. The New York diagnostic criteria are:

1. Limitation of movement of the lumbar spine in all three planes, viz. anterior flexion, lateral flexion and extension
2. History of pain (or presence of pain) at the dorsolumbar junction or in the lumbar spine
3. Limitation of chest expansion to less than 1 in. (2.5 cm) (measured at the level of the fourth intercostal space)

Ankylosing spondylitis is then considered to be definitely present if:

a) There is bilateral grade 3–4 (X-ray) sacroiliitis associated with any one clinical criterion
b) There are grade 3–4 unilateral or grade 2 bilateral radiological changes associated with criterion 1 or with both criteria 2 and 3 above.

Ankylosing spondylitis is considered to be probably present if there are grade 3–4 radiological signs alone.

These above criteria may be too rigid and might exclude mild cases or early cases in whom there may be symptoms and signs but who have not had sufficient time to express these in a radiologically visible form. Radioisotope scanning techniques may assist in the detection of such patients.

Thus the typical patient is a young male with low back pain, morning stiffness, "gelling" and limitation of spinal movement in not one but all planes. These features together allow differentiation from structural and mechanical causes of backache in which limitation of movement is in one or in a few restricted planes of movement and morning stiffness is not pronounced. Peripheral arthritis is common and may be the presenting feature. Approximately 25% of patients present with a swollen peripheral joint. The joints of the lower limb, in particular the knees, hips and ankles, are more often involved than the joints of the upper limb, and the pattern of involvement is asymmetrical. Thus the presenting complaint is often swelling of one knee or one knee together with the opposite ankle.

The pathological basis of the disease is a combination of synovitis of the diarthrodial joint and an enthesitis. The latter may be expressed as tenderness of the insertions of the great muscles around the pelvis and shoulder girdle and it is worth examining certain sites with particular care. Palpation of the nuchal crest, the insertions of the plantar aponeurosis, the iliac crests and the site of insertion of the achilles tendon may be particularly rewarding. Indeed, this may be the mode of presentation.

More frequently the disease starts in the sacroiliac joints. There is deep-seated low back pain which may radiate into the posterior aspect of thigh. Pain should not radiate below the knee and if it does so then the possibility of disc protrusion with involvement of the sciatic nerve should be considered. The disease spreads upwards and affects first the thoracic and then the cervical spine. Involvement of the costovertebral joints may produce "girdle" pains radiating around the trunk, which may produce confusion in differential diagnosis. Spread upwards into the cervical spine and the atlantoaxial joint may produce headaches which have some distinctive features. The pain begins at the back of the neck, spreads over the vertex and settles in the forehead behind the eyes. Atlantoaxial involvement with vertical or horizontal subluxation is a common and important complication of ankylosing spondylitis. Inflammatory involvement in this region may produce destruction of the stabilising transverse ligament, allowing subluxation at the odontoid peg. This and subaxial dislocation, which may be even more ominous since the diameter of the spinal canal is reduced below C-2, may produce neurological symptoms and signs either by direct pressure or by interference with local blood supply.

The pathological sequence is distinctive. The enthesitis in the spine produces inflammatory destructive changes at the corners of the vertebral bodies where the great ligaments of the spine are attached; the consequent eroded areas are called "Romanus" lesions. These damaged areas then become calcified and this is what produces the classical radiological features of the fully developed disease:

0) Normal
1) Slight narrowing of the joint space
2) Slight narrowing of the joint space plus erosions or ill-defined margins
3) Slight narrowing of the joint space plus erosions or ill-defined margins plus syndesmophytosis
4) Complete fusion of the sacroiliac joints

One feature deserves mention. On occasion an X-ray will reveal an appearance which is remarkably similar to the destruction which is caused by infection, and this can be very alarming. It may appear that one entire "mobile segment" is destroyed, and above and below this segment there are all the appearances of the bamboo spine. The pathogenesis of this lesion is interesting. The spine above and below is fused and immobile. There has been a fracture of the posterior arch, permitting movement only at this single mobile segment. The forces generated at this site during even minimal movement are immense and are responsible for the severe destruction seen on the X-ray.

Restriction of spinal movement may be documented by Schorber's test. One mark is made at the L-5/S-1 junction, one 10 cm above and another 5 cm below. The patient is then asked to flex his spine as fully as possible and the increase in distance between these marks is recorded. In passing it is important to point out that the common practice of asking the patient to touch his toes cannot be construed as a valid measure of lumbar spinal mobility. It is quite possible to achieve this using hip joint movement alone. The other measurement which is worth recording in these patients is chest expansion. This is reduced early in the course of the disease. Hip straddle provides a measure of hip joint involvement and the occiput-to-wall distance with the patient standing with his back to the wall is a measure of neck flexion. In some patients, particularly those with marked peripheral joint involvement, there may be signs of pronounced constitutional involvement, including anaemia, polymorphonuclear leucocytosis, elevated ESR and increased concentrations of all of the acute phase proteins. Serum albumin and total body weight may be reduced, mirroring this constitutional involvement. The other complications of ankylosing spondylitis are amyloidosis and rarely aortic incompetence or an unusual upper lobe fibrosis.

It has long been recognised that ankylosing spondylitis exhibits familial aggregation and the long-term follow up data generated by the Leeds unit and by Kellgren in Manchester pointed clearly to the existence of an important genetic component in the development of this disease. The description from Los Angeles and Westminster Hospital of an association between ankylosing spondylitis and the HLA-B27-containing haplotype set the seal on this and opened a Pandora's box. This work focusses attention on the "soil" and indicates that there is an immunogenetic predisposition. However, plainly only a proportion of patients with this haplotype develop the disease. Presently it is suggested that the trigger to the development of the disease is penetration of the bowel wall by one of the CREG group of organisms, possibly one of the *Klebsiella* species.

Management

One of the most important aspects of this disease is the improvement which has occurred over the past few years in management of the patient. Hitherto neglected, a great deal of attention is now focussed upon these individuals and this has transformed the prognosis. Much of the improvement is ascribable to non-drug management and the most important treatment modality is exercise. The greatest enemy of these patients is flexion and this is what must be avoided at all costs. This applies both to the axial skeleton and to the peripheral joints, and the accent must be on prevention rather than on treatment of the established and often irremediable deformity. Extension exercises must be performed several times a day and the patient should lie prone for half an hour in the morning and in the evening. The habit of swimming regularly should become part of the patient's life-style. It is important that the patient understand the purpose of all of this and the central importance of these practices to his long-term prognosis, so it is worth spending a considerable amount of time in explanation at the beginning of the illness. Time spent at this stage is time saved later. It is also important to emphasise that these patients should never be confined to bed without the most clamant reason and if this does arise then it is vital to secure the services of an experienced physiotherapist. A surprising amount of spinal mobility can be lost very quickly (i.e. within a very few weeks) and irreversibly in these circumstances. Having emphasised the vital importance of prevention it must be obvious that incipient or established flexion deformities require the most immediate and the most vigorous treatment that can be provided. Here again the help of an experienced physiotherapist is invaluable. Also, the booklets provided by such organisations as the ARC are very useful.

The second intervention technique which requires consideration is drug therapy, and the drugs concerned are described more fully in Chaps. 13 and 14. The aim should be, as always, to prescribe the minimum amount of the single drug selected on the basis of patient preference which will serve to provide the maximum relief with the minimum of adverse reactions. Ankylosing spondylitis differs slightly from rheumatoid arthritis in that the patients often have an increased rather than a reduced pain threshold and may therefore require less drug therapy. Against this, the patient is often a vigorous young male and therefore, on pharmacokinetic grounds alone, may require and tolerate a higher dose. It is also interesting that there seems to be a difference in the drugs chosen by the patient. A higher proportion of patients with this disease choose indomethacin as their preferred drug than is the case in patients with rheumatoid arthritis. Most of the remainder will select one of the other first line drugs and many will remain well controlled for many years on this regimen alone. Phenylbutazone used to be an excellent drug for patients with this disease but there are now so many safer alternatives that it should be viewed in the context of a second line drug for use in the event of failure of the primary regimen. It must be stated that the other second line drugs used in rheumatoid arthritis are ineffective and have no place in the management of these patients. Similarly, third line drugs such as corticosteroids or ACTH should be avoided. There is no place for the use of radiotherapy and no excuse in the event of the development of a malignancy or suppression of the bone marrow as a consequence of this form of intervention.

Surgical intervention may be required in the event of the development of destructive changes in the hip, where a total hip replacement may transform the patient's life and may also require to be considered in the event of the development of cervical cord damage with advancing neurological signs.

Psoriatic Arthritis

Once again, recognition of the existence of this syndrome was the result of long-term careful clinical documentation of many patients during which it became apparent that this was not simply an inconvenient variant of "sero-negative rheumatoid arthritis". The following subgroups have been identified (Wright 1981):

1. Classical psoriatic arthritis with conspicuous involvement of the distal interphalangeal joints
2. Arthritis mutilans with widespread destruction and ankylosis
3. Clinically indistinguishable from rheumatoid arthritis (without rheumatoid factor)
4. Asymmetrical oligo- or mono-arthritis
5. Psoriasis with ankylosing spondylitis

The number and composition of the subgroups may be contentious, but the separate identity of psoriatic arthritis from rheumatoid arthritis is not. This syndrome or group of syndromes belongs firmly to the seronegative spondarthritides.

Psoriatic arthritis is common and although many patients experience only mild disease, in others it may prove to be most difficult to manage. Nail changes alone, or even a family history alone, are important items of information. There is an overlap between psoriasis alone and classical ankylosing spondylitis and in addition one of the forms of psoriatic arthritis involves conspicuously the sacroiliac joints. Thus knowledge of the state of these joints is of the utmost importance. The spinal involvement may be indistinguishable from the changes which may be seen in ankylosing spondylitis, and the constitutional signs, uveitis and amyloidosis are shared complications. One form, fortunately not the most common, of peripheral joint involvement is a peculiarly destructive "arthritis mutilans" but this may also occur rarely in rheumatoid arthritis.

The presentation, evolution, complications and treatment of the dermatological manifestations are identical to those of uncomplicated psoriasis. Although often discussed, parallelism between the skin and the joint disease activity is unusual.

The relationship to MHC gene products is complicated by the separate and multiple relationships found in uncomplicated psoriasis. There is a relationship between psoriatic arthritis and the HLA-B27-containing haplotype but this is less clearly defined than in ankylosing spondylitis. The management of psoriatic arthritis differs only in detail, and especially in individual detail, from that of ankylosing spondylitis. The presence of the skin lesion may make the patient reluctant to swim regularly in a public pool. However, the principles of management and the overriding importance of regular extension exercises are identical. Although there is no evidence of an increased risk of dermatological side-effects in these patients, it seems sensible to avoid the use of a drug such as gold which is known to have the propensity to produce skin rashes.

Reiter's Syndrome [Brodie's Disease]

The triad of conjunctivitis, urethritis and arthritis was described first by Brodie and then by Hans Reiter. Perhaps in the near future this syndrome will be allocated securely to the group of diseases termed the "reactive" arthritides, but for the moment the evidence is not yet complete. There is a strong relationship to the HLA-B27 containing haplotype and it is very likely that an infection serves as the trigger. In some instances the portal of entry is probably the urogenital tract and in others the lower gastrointestinal tract, and the relationship to SARA (see above) is probably very close. One rather fortunate accident of nature has been thoroughly investigated. An outbreak of *Shigella* dysentery occurred within a closed community, namely a United States navy ship. A proportion of the sailors who were infected developed Reiter's syndrome and subsequently they were shown to possess the HLA-B27-

containing haplotype. Perhaps it would be better to discard the term Reiter's syndrome and replace it with gut-associated reactive arthritis (GARA) or SARA, specifying the responsible organism. It is likely that other members of the CREG group of organisms may act as the trigger. However, for the moment we will retain the term in common usage.

The disease occurs most commonly in the male and, although onset may be at any age, the first manifestation usually occurs in early adult life. Following an episode of urogenital or lower bowel infection the patient develops a sterile urethritis which may be accompanied by a prostatitis, conjunctivitis and an asymmetrical inflammatory polyarthritis usually affecting the lower limbs. The classical presentation is involvement of one knee together with the opposite ankle, accompanied by sacroiliitis and spondylitis. The pathology is a combination of a synovitis with enthesitis and there may be tenderness over the insertions of the tendons of the lower limb and around the pelvic girdle. The classical expression of the enthesitis is localised tenderness over the insertion of the achilles tendon or the plantar fascia. Radiologically the enthesitis is seen as exuberant fluffy calcification around the spine and the iliac crests. On X-ray of the spine there may be conspicuous, often unilateral, syndesmophytes.

Syndesmophytes are spurs of calcification arising from the margins of the vertebral bodies and growing in a vertical direction, as distinct from osteophytes which enlarge horizontally. Syndesmophytes represent calcified extensions of enthesitis of the spine, the pathological process affecting the junction of the vertebral body and the long spinal ligaments. The calcification is closely applied to the vertebral body, distinguishing this from Forrestier's disease. Syndesmophytes are found in all of the seronegative spondarthritides, reported differences between different diseases being more apparent than real. The differences between the appearances of the sacroiliac joint in the different diseases represent the spectrum of involvement rather than real differences.

There may be marked constitutional involvement, with fever, normochromic normocytic anaemia, rises in the concentration of the acute phase proteins and a high ESR. Shallow mouth ulcers are common and may be painful. A characteristic but infrequent skin manifestation is keratoderma blenorrhagicum, which is seen as a psoriatic-like eruption on the palms and soles. The elements are vesicular and pustular with scaling and lichenification. In some patients the distinction from psoriasis may be impossible and, in common with all of the members of this group, overlap syndromes are found. Thus a patient may be found to have all of the necessary criteria to make the diagnosis of Reiter's syndrome on one occasion, while at a later visit the patient may present with psoriasis, granulomatous bowel disease or classical ankylosing spondylitis. We have seen one individual who, over a period of 25 years, has suffered sequentially psoriasis, Reiter's syndrome, ankylosing spondylitis, Crohn's disease, uveitis and reactive arthritis to salmonella.

The treatment of Reiter's syndrome incorporates all of the principles of management of any chronic inflammatory polyarthritis, local treatment of the affected joints and management of complications and co-diseases. The urethritis and the conjunctivitis require only local hygiene but uveitis may be difficult to manage, necessitating local mydriatics and even corticosteroids at times.

Behçet's Syndrome

Behçet's syndrome is a combination of ocular inflammation, genital and mouth ulceration and a seronegative asymmetrical inflammatory polyarthritis. It is most common in females and clearly there is a nosological problem in some clinical situations. A patient who presents with mouth ulcers, genital inflammation, ocular inflammation and this type of polyarthritis is likely to be described as having Reiter's syndrome if male and Behçet's syndrome if female. The problem is confounded by the use of such terms as "incomplete" Reiter's or Behçet's syndrome.

Some patients will develop deep painful mouth and genital ulceration with a conspicuous and predictable relationship to menstruation and this is worth ascertaining since some of these patients may benefit from cyclical hormonal therapy. A small proportion of patients with Behçet's syndrome will develop complications which may be very serious. These include sight-threatening destructive uveitis, severe vasculitis or even pyoderma gangraenosum, and focal neurological syndromes. It must be emphasised that these are rare and there is no justification for a situation which we encountered some years ago. A 30-year-old female presented with mouth and genital ulceration and a mild polyarthritis. She had been told by a physician that she had Behçet's syndrome and that she would be dead within 2 years! Once such a story has been presented to the patient by another physician it is incredibly difficult to correct the position, and subsequent management of that patient was very difficult for several years. Of interest is the fact that the patient today is alive and well but the physician is now dead. Iatrogenesis is not confined to pharmacotherapeutics and incorrect advice may create as much havoc as any adverse drug reaction.

The management of the local ulceration rests on local measures but unlike most cases of Reiter's syndrome the ulcers of Behçet's syndrome are often very painful, requiring local anaesthetic. The management of the polyarthritis is along the usual lines. Treatment of the unusual severely affected patient may be very difficult indeed. The very number of treatments proposed for the vasculitis and the neurological syndrome testify to the individual inadequacy of each and range from transfer factor and blood transfusion on the one hand to gonadal steroids, fibrinolytic agents and heparin on the other. Some patients develop disseminated intravascular coagulation which must be managed as such. Most physicians when faced with an acutely ill and severely affected patient prescribe high dose corticosteroid.

Granulomatous Bowel Disease

Both ulcerative colitis and Crohn's disease are closely associated with this group of diseases. There is a bidirectional association of each of these with classical ankylosing spondylitis and in addition both may be associated with an asymmetrical peripheral exudative non-destructive polyarthritis. In the case of Crohn's disease and in the closely associated "blind loop" or reversed loop polyarthritis the pathogenesis has been defined. It is produced by circulating and locally deposited immune complexes and the antibody in the immune complex has activity directed against bowel organisms. The musculoskeletal diseases may precede, occur concurrently with, or succeed the bowel disorder. Amelioration of the inflammatory bowel disease may help the peripheral arthropathy, which may exhibit parallelism, but the activity and evolution of the ankylosing spondylitis proceeds independently of the bowel disorder. Management of the inflammatory bowel is along conventional lines and the local and general management of ankylosing spondylitis has been discussed. The peripheral arthritis is managed according to the principles discussed in this text. One complicating feature in the granulomatous bowel diseases is the propensity of the orally prescribed NSAIDs to affect adversely the bowel disorder and a difficult juggling act may be required to balance the impact of all of these factors in the best interests of the patient.

Further Reading

Aho K, Ahvonen P, Lassus A, Sairnen E, Sievers K, Tillikainen A (1975) HLA-B27 in reactive arthritis following infection. Ann Rheum Dis 34 [Suppl]: 29

Alexander K, Edwards C, Misko IS, Geczy AF, Bashir HV, Edmonds JP (1981) The distribution of a specific HLA-B27-associated cell surface component on the tissues of patients with ankylosing spondylitis. Clin Exp Immunol 45: 158–164

Basher HV, Geczy AF (1981) A physician's guide to HLA immunogenetics. Aust NZ J Med 11: 422–428

Calin (1981) Reiter's syndrome. In: Kelly W, Harris ED Jr, Ruddy S, Sledge CB (eds) Textbook of rheumatology, 1st edn. Saunders, Philadelphia London Toronto, Chap 65

Cudworth AG, Wolf E (1981) The HLA system and disease. Clin Sci 61: 1–5

Geczy AF, Alexander K, Bashir HV (1980) A factor(s) in *Klebsiella* culture filtrates specifically modifies an HLA-B27 associated cell surface component. Nature 238: 782–784

Good AE (1981) Enteropathic arthritis. In: Kelly W, Harris ED Jr, Ruddy S, Sledge CB (eds) Textbook of rheumatology, 1st edn. Saunders, Philadelphia London Toronto, Chap 67

Keat AC, Maini RN, Pegrum GD, Scott JT (1979) The clinical features and HLA associations of reactive arthritis associated with non-gonococcal urethritis. Q J Med 48: 323–342

Moll JMH (1981) Ankylosing spondylitis. Churchill Livingstone, Edinburgh London New York

O'Duffy JD (1981) Behçet's disease. In: Kelly W, Harris ED Jr, Ruddy S, Sledge CB (eds) Textbook of rheumatology, 1st edn. Saunders, Philadelphia London Toronto, Chap 74

Winblad S (1975) Arthritis associated with *Yersinia enterocolitica* infections. Scan J Infect Dis 7: 191–195

Wright V (1978) Seronegative polyarthritis. Arthritis Rheum 21: 619–633

Wright V, Chamberlain MA (1979) Behçet's syndrome. Bull Rheum Dis 29: 972–977

Wright V (1981) Psoriatic arthritis. In: Kelly W, Harris ED Jr, Ruddy S, Sledge CB (eds) Textbook of rheumatology, 1st edn. Saunders, Philadelphia London Toronto, Chap 66

11 Infective Arthritis and Polymyalgia Rheumatica/Giant Cell Arteritis

Introduction

Despite the variety of organisms which are responsible for infecting bones and joints, the possible responses to these agents by the host is limited and hence the symptoms and signs of an infective arthritis are relatively stereotyped (Table 11.1). Where differences do occur they are differences in emphasis rather than in basic pathophysiology.

Table 11.1. Mechanisms of tissue damage (modified from Platt and Dick 1982)

Type	Characteristics	Examples
1) Direct infection	Multiplication of organism in joint	Pyogenic arthritis Tuberculosis
2) Post-infective	Presence of microbial antigen within joint	Hepatitis B Postmeningococcal
3) Cross-reactive	Infection elsewhere but neither organism nor antigen in joint	Rheumatic fever Cross-reacting enteropathic Gram-negative bacilli, e.g. Yersinia
4) Inductive "Self+X"	Modification of host cell by organism	? Rheumatoid Seronegative spondarthritides

Acute Pyogenic Arthritis

The incidence of pyogenic arthritis has fallen during the past 30 years, and there have been changes in the age distribution. Whereas acute pyogenic arthritis was characteristically a disease of childhood, the emphasis is now

shifting towards an older age group and to patients with underlying diseases.
A "red hot joint" is a medical emergency and demands prompt
aspiration. The major differential diagnoses are sepsis or a crystal-induced
synovitis and the only certain method to discriminate between these two
important possibilities is examination of synovial fluid. In the case of a
septic arthritis, thick pus requiring a wide-bore needle for aspiration is often
present.

The agent responsible for the majority of cases of acute pyogenic arthritis
seen in Britain is *Staphylococcus aureus*. Other organisms which may be
responsible include haemolytic streptococcus, pneumococcus, *E. coli*,
salmonella, pseudomonas, *Haemophilus influenzae*, bacteroides and others.
Both staphylococci and salmonella show a predilection to involve the hip
joint.

The histological appearances of an acute pyogenic arthritis are
characteristic, with pronounced polymorphonuclear leucocyte infiltrate,
oedema and necrosis. Infection can reach a joint by haematogenous spread,
by local extension from pre-existing infection in soft tissue or bone and
occasionally by accidental or therapeutic direct puncture. If the diagnosis is
delayed or treatment is inadequate or inappropriate, very severe tissue
destruction can occur and the morbidity and even mortality rise in
proportion to time taken to institute effective treatment.

Radiological changes in the acute stage are absent unless there is pre-
existing damage. However, destruction of articular cartilage and changes in
underlying bone may be seen after a few weeks. The increasing availability
of radioisotopic techniques offers a hope for earlier diagnosis.

The consequences of infection in children can be particularly severe in
view of the possible damage to the epiphysis with subsequent deformity.
Furthermore the vascular anatomy of the hip joint in the young child in
which terminal end arteries penetrate the head of the femur provides an
additional route of infection.

Acute pyogenic arthritis may occur in patients with pre-existing joint
disease, in particular in patients with rheumatoid arthritis, and may be
mistaken for an exacerbation of the underlying disorder. Patients with
immunosuppression due to disease or treatment are liable to develop
pyogenic arthritis, which may be due to unusual organisms such as the
bacterioides. The clinical signs and symptoms normally associated with the
presence of sepsis may be masked by immunosuppression or disease, leading
to late recognition of the problem and hence severe damage.

Patients who have undergone prosthetic joint surgery are at risk from a
variety of organisms. Infection may lead to failure of the prosthesis due to
loosening of the cement and force removal of the prosthesis before the
infection can be controlled. Prosthetic infection may occur early
postoperatively or alternatively may emerge only many years later. In the
late infections the organisms involved nevertheless may still prove to have
been introduced at the original operation. Persistent infection may lead to
the formation of a fistula which may prove difficult to eradicate despite
vigorous antibiotic treatment.

Osteomyelitis may occur in association with pyogenic infection by direct spread from an infected joint or vice versa. Sympathetic effusions, which are sterile, may occur in association with osteomyelitis and may produce diagnostic confusion.

In addition to causing damage in the appendicular skeleton, pyogenic infections affect the axial skeleton. In particular the vertebrae and sacroiliac joints may be infected by *Staphylococcus aureus*.

Gonococcal Infections

The incidence of gonococcal arthritis has risen with the increased incidence of gonococcal infections in the population, although the increase in Britain has been much less marked than in the U.S.A. The disease is more common in females than males, as females are the major reservoir of untreated gonococcal infection in the population. There are two mechanisms by which gonococcal infections produce joint involvement; firstly, a direct type 1 acute purulent arthritis and secondly, a type 3 reactive arthritis.

The clinical picture of polyarthralgia tenosynovitis, fever and skin lesions is characteristic. The joints most commonly involved are the knee, wrist and small joints of the hand, with polyarticular involvement being more common than monoarticular. The skin lesions usually begin as red papules that either disappear or proceed through vesicular and pustular stages.

The rise in the incidence of urethritis has led to an increased incidence of sexually acquired reactive arthritis (SARA), which is associated with the presence of the HLA-B27 haplotype.

Brucella Infections

As the incidence of brucella infection has fallen, bone and joint involvement have become uncommon. Various patterns of infection can occur: a monoarthritis, a bursitis (particularly pretibial bursitis) and most characteristically spondylitis. This may develop weeks or months after infection and may present as severe back pain. Radiology shows a destructive lesion with narrowing of the disc space, and characteristically there is associated exuberant osteophyte formation.

Tuberculosis

The incidence of tuberculosis involving bones and joints has fallen under the triple onslaught of better general conditions of hygiene and nutrition, preventive measures and effective chemotherapy. Despite this it still occurs, particularly in some immigrant groups and the elderly, and may be missed through failure to include it as a possible differential diagnosis. The most commonly affected site is the thoracic spine, where involvement of a vertebral body leads to production of a cavity filled with caseous material. Extension frequently occurs to the intervertebral disc, which is characteristically destroyed, and to other vertebrae.

A severe deformity may develop at this site, with marked angulation leading to the formation of a gibbus deformity and cord compression. Paravertebral abscesses may form secondary to vertebral involvement and may track along tissue planes to produce the classical psoas abscess. Sacroiliac joint involvement occurs and should be considered, particularly when the sacroiliitis is unilateral. The appendicular skeleton may also be affected by tuberculosis. Children rarely develop a dactylitis, which may be associated with tenosynovitis.

Any large joint can be involved by tuberculosis, the hip and knee being most frequently involved, with symptoms of gradual loss of movement, swelling, stiffness and pain. Tuberculous synovitis may require a formal open biopsy before a diagnosis can be made on the basis of the characteristic histological findings of caseating granulomata.

Syphilitic Infections

Bone and joint involvement may occur in both congenital and acquired forms. In the congenital form osteochondritis, periostitis and, rarely, dactylitis occur. Clutton's joints present as intermittent non-inflammatory knee joint effusions. Acquired forms include a variety of lesions: periostitis, gummata and in the tertiary stages of neurosyphilis, neuropathic or Charcot's joints. Charcot's joints may yield synovial fluid containing free and ingested crystals of calcium pyrophosphate dihydrate.

Rheumatic Fever

Acute rheumatic fever is now very rare in the developed countries but still occurs frequently in the third world. The clinical features of carditis, flitting polyarthritis, nodules, chorea and erythema marginatum are well known. The joints are warm and swollen with erythema, particularly over the smaller joints. Erythema marginatum, although characteristic, only occurs in a small proportion of active cases and then only fleetingly. The characteristic feature is the sharply demarcated spreading edge of the lesion.

During the present discussions revolving around the concept of "reactive" arthritis, it is often forgotten that rheumatic fever represents the original and still arguably the most secure model of this process in man.

Viral Arthritis

Self-limiting polyarthritides are being recognised increasingly in association with common viral infections such as rubella and infectious mononucleosis. Joint symptoms occur in only a small proportion of cases in these infections; however, a much higher frequency is reported in the arthropod-borne viral diseases such as Chikungunya and O'Nyong-Nyong. Instead of polymorphonuclear leucocytes as in rheumatoid arthritis, the synovial fluid in viral arthritides contains a preponderance of monocytic cells.

Of a more controversial nature is the role of viruses in the induction of chronic destructive inflammatory arthritides such as rheumatoid arthritis, where one outcome of interaction between viral nucleic acid and host DNA may be modification of the host cells. Certainly there has been a resurgence of interest in the past decade in the interaction of exogenous infection with an immunogenetically predisposed host.

By far the most important step in the management of a patient with an infective arthritis is prompt diagnosis and the earliest possible institution of appropriate drug treatment. Both the types of offending organisms and the appropriate antibiotic change so quickly and vary so greatly in different areas that it would be futile and potentially dangerous to provide a list of suggestions. It is better to stress the importance of early and definitive diagnosis and the urgent need to work closely with local bacteriological colleagues. Depending upon the circumstances either closed or open continuous drainage may be required. In the latter event the assistance of local orthopaedic colleagues is essential.

Once appropriate antibacterial treatment has been instituted and as soon as it is clear that the patient is responding then it is time to consider optimum rehabilitation programmes. From the outset the affected joint should have been splinted in the position of optimum future function. As soon as is practicable a programme of carefully graduated exercises for the affected area and for all other muscle groups must be initiated.

Polymyalgia Rheumatica and Giant Cell Arteritis

This is an interesting inflammatory syndrome which fits neither with rheumatoid arthritis nor with the seronegative arthritides. It does bear some relationship to the vasculitides and the multisystem disorders; hence it can conveniently be discussed at this juncture.

The diagnostic criteria for polymyalgia rheumatica and giant cell arthritis are listed below.

Polymyalgia rheumatica
1. Shoulder and pelvic girdle muscle pain without weakness
2. Pronounced and distinct morning stiffness
3. Duration of 2 months (unless treated)
4. ESR over 30
5. Absence of other defined rheumatic, malignant, hepatic or neuromuscular disease
6. Prompt (within 1 week) response to prednisolone

Giant cell arteritis
1. Disturbance of vision
2. Tenderness over the temporal artery
3. Histological changes in temporal artery biopsy
4. Involvement of other muscular medium-sized arteries. N.B. Carotid, brachial, radial, renal, femoral and popliteal arteries *must* be examined in every case.
5. Clinical features pointing to involvement of other vessels and to constitutional disease including jaw claudication, severe headaches, cerebrovascular signs, unexplained normochromic normocytic anaemia, weight loss and depression

Aches and pains with some degree of stiffness are common complaints in the elderly and the additional symptoms of feeling tired and depressed too easily may be accepted as part of growing old. It is important to remember the concept of the "elderly elite". This stems from the work of Professor Ferguson Anderson in Glasgow, who focussed attention on a group of octogenarians in whom all physical and mental faculties were intact, the vascular tree was normal and there was no evidence of arthritis. The calendar age of these patients did not mirror their biological age and it was emphasised that these people must be approached in all respects in the context of the latter and not the former figure.

However, in some patients these same symptoms referred to above may herald the onset of an important rheumatic disease which is more common than is often supposed. Polymyalgia rheumatica is a disease of the elderly commonly affecting patients over the age of 60 years. The most important symptom is severe stiffness, particularly in the morning, affecting the shoulder and pelvic girdle. This may be so severe that the patient is unable to rise from bed in the morning and has to roll over to get up. Pain is usually overshadowed by the complaint of stiffness and there may be conspicuous signs of constitutional upset with fatigue, weakness, fever, anaemia, arthralgia and severe depression. Weight loss may be so pronounced that it is common to inherit a patient who has been thoroughly investigated for malignancy, and the anaemia may be the presenting feature.

The most significant investigation and the simplest is the ESR, which is usually elevated, often markedly to values in excess of 100 mm/hour. Other investigations including muscle biopsy and X-ray of joints are usually unhelpful and the anaemia is normochromic and normocytic.

This syndrome may be "primary" in the sense that there may be no discernible underlying pathology. In other patients, however, it may mark the onset of another disease such as rheumatoid arthritis, chronic liver disease, malignancy or myeloma, and this is where the greatest problems arise. In the primary form a proportion of patients will develop giant cell arteritis, emphasising the importance of palpating and auscultating all major vessels as a routine in all such patients. Alternatively some patients who present with giant cell arteritis will subsequently develop polymyalgia rheumatica although this is less common, particularly today when most patients with giant cell arteritis are treated with corticosteroids.

Giant cell arteritis affects those extracranial arteries which possess an internal elastic lamina. The patient presents with headache, claudicant pain on chewing and scalp tenderness which may be so severe that the patient can no longer wear a hat. Involvement of the vertebrobasilar artery may produce ischaemic brain stem syndromes, but the most significant vascular involvement is the ophthalmic artery. Blindness may develop suddenly with no warning or there may be warning visual symptoms such as flashing lights or fortification spectra. Approximately 10% of these patients become blind and it is estimated that 240 persons on the blind register in England and Wales owe their blindness to this condition.

The diagnosis may be confirmed by arterial biopsy, with or without preliminary arteriography. The histological appearance is distinctive, with disruption of the vessel wall and internal elastic lamina, infiltration with white cells and the presence of giant cells. Biopsy is often positive in patients who apparently have polymyalgia alone, and in patients presenting with temporal arteritis the presence of tenderness of the vessel wall correlates closely with positivity on biopsy. Certainly it is more important to examine for tenderness and to treat immediately on suspicion rather than to wait for the result of the biopsy. Treatment for a few days with corticosteroid does not alter the appearances on biopsy, so the priority is to treat and to arrange the biopsy as soon as possible thereafter.

Prednisolone is the treatment of choice both for polymyalgia, when a dose of less than 10 mg per day is usually adequate, and for temporal arteritis, in which case it is important to start with much higher doses (60 mg per day). Only the higher dose will protect from blindness. It is rarely necessary nor advisable to maintain this high dose, but response to prednisolone in both diseases is so dramatic and so fast that absence of response within 1 week should throw doubt upon the initial diagnosis. The maintenance dose should at all times be the lowest possible dose consistent with response as judged by symptoms, signs and the ESR.

Further Reading

Behn AR, Mathews JA, Phillip I (1978) Lactate UV system; a rapid method for the diagnosis of septic arthritis. Ann Rheum Dis 40: 489–492

Borenstein DG, Gibbs CA, Jacobs RP (1982) Gas-liquid chromatographic analysis of synovial fluid. Arthritis Rheum 25: 947–953

Chantler JK, Ford DK, Tingle AJ (1982) Persistent rubella infection and rubella associated arthritis. Lancet I: 1323–1325

Greenwood BM, Whittle HC (1976) The pathogenesis of meningococcal arthritis. In: Dumonde DC (ed) Infection and immunology in the rheumatic diseases. Blackwell, Oxford, pp 119–127

Hallidie-Smith KA, Bywaters EGL (1958) The differential diagnosis of rheumatic fever. Arch Dis Child 33: 350–358

Hunder GG, Hazleman BL (1981) Giant cell arteritis and polymyalgia rheumatica. In: Kelly W, Harris ED Jr, Ruddy S, Sledge CB (eds) Textbook of rheumatology, 1st edn. Saunders, Philadelphia London Toronto, Chap 73

Huston KA, Hunder GG, Lie JT, Kennedy PH, Elveback LR (1978) Temporal arteritis; a 25 year epidemiologic, clinic and pathologic study. Ann Intern Med 82(2): 162–168

Mitchell WS, Brooks PM, Stevenson RD, Buchanan WW (1976) Septic arthritis in patients with rheumatoid arthritis; a still underdiagnosed complication. J Rheumatol 3: 124–130

Mowatt AG (1979) Generalised rheumatism, polymyalgia rheumatica and its differential diagnosis. Saunders, London Philadelphia Toronto (Clin Rheum Dis, vol 5, pp 775–781)

Mulley GP (1982) Giant cell arteritis. Medicine 27: 413–416

Park JR, Jones JG, Hazelman BL (1981) Relationship of the erythrocyte sedimentation rate to acute phase proteins in polymyalgia rheumatica and giant cell arteritis. Ann Rheum Dis 40: 493–495

Shipley M (1978) Infection and arthritis. Saunders, London Philadelphia Toronto (Clin Rheum Dis, vol 4)

12 Connective Tissue Disorders

Introduction

This is a difficult and controversial area where the exotic may fascinate to deceive. Ironically patients with one of the more common chronic arthritides are often neglected while patients with equally incurable but rare connective tissue disorders may suffer from a surfeit of attention. Thus patients with one of the multisystem diseases such as SLE are often overinvestigated, overdoctored and overtreated.

Diagnosis

A precise diagnosis may be difficult and this initial obstacle bewilders and frustrates the clinician. There is a strong temptation to force symptoms and signs to conform to a preconceived diagnosis; the next step is to introduce heroic therapy thought appropriate for that diagnosis and gross mismanagement may result. Acute, rapidly progressive presentations are the exception, and a conservative approach can be adopted in most cases. Some diagnoses eventually become apparent only over a period of months or years and prolonged follow up with careful documentation is most important. For much of the time the clinician will be treating clusters of symptoms and signs and a label may be only of academic interest.

Biochemical and serological tests should not be viewed in isolation in these patients. As always, there is no substitute for painstaking clinical assessment. Where a firm diagnosis cannot be reached, frank discussion with the patient is necessary while emphasising the benign nature of many symptoms. Equally, if a diagnosis is reached, education of the patient and family, discussion, and re-evaluation are mandatory. The nature of the disease may alter radically over a period of years and a formal review of diagnosis can be most helpful. This should aim to be comprehensive but investigations, particularly invasive tests, should not be repeated unnecessarily. It is not the purpose of this text to review the aetiology, pathogenesis or clinical features of these diseases, and we have provided a bibliography at the end of this chapter for readers who wish to pursue these areas.

Approach to Management

Chekov commented in the *Cherry Orchard* "when a lot of remedies are suggested for a disease that means it can't be cured". This comment is unfortunately applicable to many of the connective tissue disorders and needs to be acknowledged at the outset. Nevertheless, amelioration is possible, and a positive approach vital.

Unhurried explanation, education and reassurance of the patient and family may obviate the need for chemotherapy in mild disease and diminish the requirement in moderate disease. Precise strategy must be tailored to the individual patient and disease, and frequent consultation may be necessary. These patients are often extremely anxious and fragmentary management of multisystem disease may exacerbate this anxiety still further. Continuity is vital, and the team approach every bit as necessary as for the patient with rheumatoid arthritis. The presence of a team member well acquainted with a case history will often save needless investigation, admission or treatment. Experienced observers tend to be more cautious therapists in this sphere, sometimes to the point of therapeutic nihilism.

There might be a case for referral to specialised centres where experimental therapy, if used, should form part of a controlled study. In this way solutions may ultimately be found for the many unanswered questions. Few adequately controlled trials of therapy have been carried out, mainly because diverse manifestations and small numbers in any one clinic necessitate multicentre studies with all their attendant problems.

The remainder of this discussion will deal with the management of connective tissue disorders in two ways:

1. Treatment of symptoms and signs common to a number of diseases will be outlined.
2. Features peculiar to particular diseases will be discussed within the framework of each entity.

Management of Symptoms and Signs

Raynaud's Phenomenon

The single most useful measure in the management of Raynaud's phenomenon is avoidance of cold. Advice about the role of cigarettes and stress should be given, but patients are rarely amenable to the necessary changes in life-style. Surgical sympathectomy was at one time widely practiced but gives at best temporary benefit and is no longer recommended.

While symptomatic benefit is clearly of importance to the sufferer, most patients with Raynaud's phenomenon cope if able to avoid extreme cold and if reassured about the usually benign course of the complaint. The problem of severe Raynaud's phenomenon complicated by painful digital ulcers is more urgent. Many treatments have been tried—some in an attempt to diminish sympathetic activity, others with a rheological or immunological approach. The extensive list includes guanethidine, methyldopa, tolazoline, phenoxybenzamine, prazosin, reserpine, griseofulvin, stanozolol, prostacyclin, plasma exchange and behaviour therapy. To date none of these has been of proven sustained benefit, and variation in disease activity and in climatic conditions makes scientific assessment a difficult exercise.

Polyarthropathy

Polyarthralgia is a feature of many connective tissue disorders and may progress to frank arthritis (which is, however, usually non-erosive). Nevertheless, deformity may result from tendinous involvement, and general preventive measures such as splinting should be implemented where necessary. Symptomatic non-steroidal anti-inflammatory drugs should be used intermittently as required. The advisability of surgical intervention needs careful consideration; cosmetic expectations are not realistic, but procedures such as stabilisation of the interphalangeal joint of the thumb (when subject to recurrent dislocation) may be useful. It is important to be aware of the possibility of joint infection, which may rapidly prove fatal. Aseptic necrosis may occur and may require major joint replacement. Corticosteroid therapy is seldom indicated for joint symptoms.

Alopecia

This is a feature of both SLE and progressive systemic sclerosis (PSS) which is difficult to treat and which patients find most distressing. Alopecia does not respond predictably to any therapy but often improves as the general activity of the disease diminishes. Reassurance is necessary, along with appropriate advice about a wig. Occasionally cytotoxic therapy in itself will produce hair fall which reverses on cessation of therapy.

Myopathy

Myalgia is a common complaint in many rheumatological disorders, and before embarking on therapy it is important that a positive diagnosis of myositis be made. Where muscle enzyme, EMG and biopsy studies confirm the clinical diagnosis, corticosteroids are generally considered the drug of choice (although again there are no controlled studies). Very large doses are not necessarily indicated, and attempts to reduce the dose gradually or to change to an alternate day regimen should be made. Occasionally the addition of a cytotoxic drug such as azathioprine cyclophosphamide or methotrexate may be required to control disease activity or to act as a steroid-sparing agent. Careful monitoring of muscle strength and, in some severe cases, of respiratory function, is necessary. The aim should be to keep the patient mobile, but complete return to clinical and biochemical normality is seldom attained. Steroid myopathy may complicate assessment of response.

Serositis

Pericarditis, pleuritis or peritonitis may occur in many connective tissue disorders and exclusion of infection or pulmonary thromboembolism is essential. Simple therapeutic measures such as indomethacin should be tried first. Corticosteroid therapy is seldom indicated for serositis in the absence of other visceral involvement.

Other Cardiac and Pulmonary Manifestations

Myocarditis is difficult to recognise but when diagnosed is probably an indication for corticosteroid therapy. There is no effective treatment for diffuse pneumonitis or fibrosing alveolitis, but attention must be paid to episodes of infection. Oxygen will be needed in severe cases.

Fever

Pyrexial episodes may occur during the course of connective tissue disorders and differentiation of disease activity from infection is difficult. Repeated diligent searches for sepsis or septic foci should be carried out and the possible coexistence of disease flare and infection must be borne in mind. It has been suggested that C-reactive protein is of value in differentiation in SLE patients (being elevated in septic episodes but not when disease is active).

Hypertension

Meticulous control of hypertension, whether it occurs in SLE, PSS or PAN (polyarteritis nodosa) is mandatory. This is a positive contribution which can and must be made to reduce morbidity and mortality in the patient with connective tissue disease. Drug therapy with steroids or NSAID may contribute to a rise in blood pressure.

Arteritis

Classification of arteritis represents one of the most bewildering aspects of modern rheumatology, and this brief discussion makes no pretensions. It is purely pragmatic and no philosophy is attempted.

Giant cell arteritis is considered by most clinicians as an imperative indication for corticosteroids. The dose should be sufficient to control symptoms and reduce the ESR. Careful long-term monitoring is vital.

Vasculitis of the polyarteritis nodosa and Wegener's granulomatosis group is often severe and life threatening. Corticosteroids alone in this setting have proved disappointing, but encouraging results have been reported using cyclophosphamide. Again, pretreatment assessment should be thorough and close follow-up with tailoring of the dose is necessary.

Arteritis occurring in the course of rheumatoid arthritis can be most difficult to manage. Digital vasculitis in itself usually needs no therapy. Corticosteroids are usually prescribed in varying dose, but it is possible that sudden change in the dose may itself precipitate vasculitis. The role of plasma exchange with or without concurrent prescription of cytotoxic drugs remains a matter for speculation.

Features Particular to Different Diagnostic Groups

Systemic Lupus Erythematosus

In addition to the features discussed above, some manifestations of SLE are virtually peculiar to this disease and will be considered here. As in all chronic disease the approach to the SLE patient needs time and repeated visits to reassess and discuss the disease, and frequent reassurance. Do not treat laboratory results in isolation. Very acute multisystem presentations are rare but should obviously be treated promptly and vigorously. In such a circumstance with evidence of advancing visceral involvement, few would argue that the drug of choice is prednisolone, initially in high doses (over 60 mg per day). Always think of infection if unexplained deterioration occurs in an SLE patient.

Photosensitivity

Sensible avoidance of sun exposure along with appropriate protective clothing will do much to diminish morbidity from photosensitivity in SLE. The prophylactic use of a sun screen cream such as mexenone 4% or padimate 2.5% (alcoholic solution) offers protection where some UV radiation is unavoidable. Patient compliance is important here, and careful explanation of the aims of therapy is necessary.

Skin Rash

Topical treatment of the rash of SLE is often disappointing. Chloroquine may be indicated where cutaneous features predominate rather than visceral involvement. Ophthalmological monitoring is mandatory.

Neuropsychiatric Disorders

Many SLE patients appear anxious and the majority require repeated reassurance and psychological support over the course of their disease. Overt neurological symptoms and signs may improve spontaneously, and active intervention is not always indicated. In the acute phase of CNS lupus, high dose steroid (60–80 mg) has been advocated but equally a case has been made for conservative management with admission to hospital, bed rest and close observation. Whichever course is followed (and there is no controlled data to act as a guide), exclusion of underlying infection should always be the priority. The danger of opportunistic infection in patients on high dose steroid is considerable.

The differentiation of corticosteroid-induced psychosis from acute cerebral lupus can be difficult but this possibility should also be borne in mind. If anticonvulsants are required then these must be monitored most carefully and it must be remembered that they may induce liver enzymes and increase the metabolism of corticosteroid. In patients who have long-standing epilepsy and develop evidence of SLE, drug-induced disease should be considered. There is no documented additional risk in prescribing anticonvulsant therapy in patients with known SLE and convulsions. They are probably not needed after only one uncomplicated seizure.

Judicious use of antidepressants or major tranquillisers may allow reduction of steroid dose although controlled data are again not available.

Intractable headaches may be a feature of active SLE and in the absence of infection no specific therapy is of proven benefit.

Renal Disease

Treatment of renal disease is one of the most controversial aspects of SLE management. Renal biopsy appearances may change over the course of the disease and are not a foolproof guide. Most physicians would give no therapy for minimal change disease, but monitoring of urinary sediment and protein should continue. In the face of the nephrotic syndrome or of diffuse proliferative glomerulonephritis, corticosteroids with or without cytotoxics are often given. Yet again controlled data are not available, but if corticosteroids are used the general principles of using the minimum dose and trying alternate day regimens should be applied. Similarly, the least toxic immunosuppressive should be tried, azathioprine probably being the most appropriate. Attention should be paid to treatment of intercurrent infection, to the control of hypertension and to general supportive measures. The use of plasmaphoresis and bolus high dose methyl prednisolone is experimental.

Whatever the therapeutic intervention selected, it is mandatory to monitor response carefully and quantitatively. If there has been no response within a reasonable time (less than 1 month) then the therapy must be withdrawn to avoid the accumulation of ineffective yet hideously toxic regimes.

Haematological Manifestations

Anaemia. Normochromic normocytic anaemia does not respond to oral iron but often improves during periods of disease remission. Severe haemolytic anaemia is unusual but may necessitate corticosteroid therapy.

Leucopenia. No specific therapy is usually required, but cytotoxic drugs, if used for other reasons, will need very careful monitoring. Lithium may exert an effect but this is usually transient. If the neutrophil count drops to below 1000 cells per mm^3 then the patient will be very likely to develop a potentially life-threatening infection and barrier nursing should be instituted together with prophylactic antibiotics. Cell transfusions may be required.

Thrombocytopenia. Very low platelet counts or moderate depression along with symptoms or signs of bleeding will also require corticosteroid. Splenectomy may be required in certain circumstances.

Drug Reactions

The list of drugs possibly implicated in causing an SLE-like syndrome are as follows:

1. *Drugs definitely implicated*:
Procainamide
Hydralazine
Isoniazid
2. *Drugs probably implicated*:
Chlorpromazine
Methyldopa
Phenytoins
Penicillamine
Quinidine
Propyl thiouracil
Lithium carbonate
Nitrofurantoin
Some β-blockers
3. *Drugs possibly implicated*:
Griseofulvin
Sulphonamides
Penicillin
Oral contraceptives

The similarity of this syndrome to natural SLE has been overstressed and it should be emphasised that most adverse reactions of this type are heralded by the appearance of antinuclear factor in serum (but not by a positive Farr test) and remit promptly and completely on withdrawal of the offending agent.

Many patients with idiopathic SLE will tolerate oral contraceptives, and while exacerbations have been reported in patients receiving oestrogens of any kind, cause and effect are difficult to establish with these commonly prescribed compounds. Sulphonamides are probably best avoided, and antituberculous therapy should be instituted with close observation. There is no firm evidence that hydralazine, procainamide or phenytoins will exacerbate idiopathic SLE but where a satisfactory alternative is available it seems reasonable to use it.

Fatigue

Non-specific complaints of fatigue are found in all patients at some stage of their disease and do not necessarily correlate well with objective evidence of disease activity. No specific treatment is available but reassurance and advice about adequate rest and avoidance of stress are important.

Pregnancy

An increased tendency to spontaneous abortion and to disease flare in the puerperium is reported in SLE. It does not, however, seem reasonable to advise patients who are keen to have children against pregnancy unless there is severe cardiac, pulmonary or renal disease. Barrier methods of contraception may be preferable to an IUD or contraceptive pill but may be unacceptable to some patients.

Progressive Systemic Sclerosis

Skin

There is no therapy of proven benefit in the skin changes of PSS. It has been suggested that in the early stages penicillamine may have a role, and that corticosteroids may provide transient benefit in patients who have a marked inflammatory cell infiltrate on biopsy. Neither of these claims has been substantiated and both therapies are hazardous in the long term. Adequate warmth and scrupulous attention to skin sepsis may provide amelioration. Similarly, bland creams which combat skin dryness may prove beneficial.

Dysphagia

There is no effective therapy for dysphagia. Dietary advice about texture of food, fluid intake and posture should be given. Symptomatic treatment for oesophagitis or stricture may be necessary. Stasis may lead to bacterial overgrowth and malabsorption and appropriate antibiotic therapy should be given.

Renal Involvement

There is again no specific therapy, but hypertension should be carefully controlled. Since the extent and the progression of renal involvement so often become the critical factor in the later stages of this disease it is very important to monitor renal function carefully throughout the course of the disease. This may be achieved by regular estimations of serum creatinine.

Recently it has been suggested that the converting enzyme inhibitor "captopril" may be worth considering in the patient with hypertension and renal involvement. PSS patients have undergone renal transplantations and in some of these patients recurrences of the disease have been documented.

Conclusion

It is striking how much more time patients with rare connective tissue disorders demand in the clinic or ward. Their handicap may not be as overt as that of the rheumatoid patient—indeed, in many instances objective evaluation will show minimal abnormality—yet these patients are often exceptionally anxious and lengthy discussion and reassurance may be required. In addition, amongst this group will be an acutely ill minority with life-threatening disease where prompt assessment and treatment is indicated. Thus the demands on resources may be extensive and are likely to be disproportionate to the numbers of patients involved.

It is striking that patients with diseases such as SLE who live their lives in temperate climates such as the United Kingdom seem to be affected much less severely than patients who live in warmer climes. This raises many interesting questions about the influences of race and sunshine upon the disease but in addition it carries its own message for patient management. Many patients in Britain can be managed by reassurance, and corticosteroids are required less often and in lower doses than is the case in the Southern states of North America or in the Middle East.

Further Reading

Adams RD (1975) Diseases of muscle, 3rd edn. Harper and Row, Hagerstown Maryland New York Evanston San Francisco London

Appenzeller O, Williams RC (1979) Cerebral lupus erythematosus. Ann Intern Med 90: 430–431

Chumbley LC, Harrison EG Jr, DeReme RA (1977) Allergic granulomatosis and angiitis (Churg-Strauss syndrome). Report and analysis of 30 cases. Mayo Clin Proc 52: 477

Decker JL, Steinberg AD, Reinersten JL, Plotz PH, Balow JE, Klippel JH (1979) Systemic lupus erythematosus; evolving concepts. Ann Intern Med 91: 587–604

Dubois EL (1974) Lupus erythematosus. A review of the current status of discoid and systemic lupus erythematosus and their variants, 2nd edn. University of Southern California Press, Los Angeles

Editorial (1982) Monitoring of SLE. Lancet II: 251

Fauci AS, Katz P, Haynes BF, Wolff SM (1979) Cyclophosphamide therapy of severe systemic necrotising vasculitis. N Engl J Med 301: 235–238

Goodman WS and Gilman AC (eds) (1980) The pharmacological basis of therapeutics, 6th edn. Macmillan, New York Toronto London

Graham JR (1981) Localised systemic sclerosis. In: Kelly W, Harris ED Jr, Ruddy S, Sledge CB (eds) Textbook of rheumatology, 1st edn. Saunders, Philadelphia London Toronto, Chap 78

Griffiths IDG, Dick WC (1979) Antibodies to DNA antigens; their specificity and clinical relevance. Eur J Clin Invest 9: 239–241

Hess EV (1981) Introduction to drug-related lupus. Arthritis Rheum 24: 6–9

Hughes GRV (1979) Connective tissue disorders. Blackwell Scientific Publications, Oxford

Hunder GG, Conn DL (1981) Necrotising vasculitis. In: Kelly W, Harris ED Jr, Ruddy S, Sledge CB (eds) Textbook of rheumatology, 1st edn. Saunders, Philadelphia London Toronto, Chap 72

Kauffman RH, Herrman WA, Meyer CJLM, Daha MR, Van Es LA (1980) Circulating IgA immune complexes in Henoch-Schönlein purpura. J Med 69: 859–866

Marx WJ, O'Connell DJ (1979) Arthritis of primary biliary cirrhosis. Arch Intern Med 139: 213–216

Reynolds TB, Denison EK, Frankl HD, Lieberman HL, Peters RL (1971) Primary biliary cirrhosis with scleroderma, Raynaud's phenomenon and telangiectasia. Am J Med 50: 302–312

Reza MJ, Dornfield L, Goldberg LS, Bluestone R, Pearson CM (1975) Wegener's granulomatosis; long term follow up of patients treated with cyclophosphamide. Arthritis Rheum 18: 501–505

Rodnan GP (1979) Progressive systemic sclerosis. Saunders, Philadelphia London Toronto (Clin Rheum Dis, vol 5/1)

Rothfield N (ed) (1975) Systemic lupus erythematosus. Saunders, Philadelphia London Toronto (Clin Rheum Dis, vol 1)

Rothfield N (1981) Clinical features of SLE. In: Kelly W, Harris ED Jr, Ruddy S, Sledge CB (eds) Textbook of rheumatology, 1st edn. Saunders, Philadelphia London Toronto, Chap 69

Sharp GC (1981) Mixed connective tissue disease and overlap syndromes. In: Kelly W, Harris ED Jr, Ruddy S, Sledge CB (eds) Textbook of rheumatology, 1st edn. Saunders, Philadelphia London Toronto, Chap 71

Sharp GC, Irvine WS, Tan EM, Gould RG, Holman HR (1972) Mixed connective tissue disease—an apparently distinct rheumatic disease syndrome associated with a specific antibody to an extractable nuclear antigen (E.N.A.). Am J Med 52: 148–159

Shulman LE (1977) Diffuse fasciitis with eosinophilia; a new syndrome. Arthritis Rheum 20: 205–15

Steinberg AD (1981) Management of S.L.E. In: Kelly W, Harris ED Jr, Ruddy S, Sledge CB (eds) Textbook of rheumatology, 1st edn. Saunders, Philadelphia London Toronto, Chap 70

Swaak AJG, Groenwold J, Aarden LA, Statius Van Eps LW, Feltkamp TEW (1982) Prognostic value of anti-ds DNA in SLE. Ann Rheum Dis 41: 388–395

Velayos EE, Masi AT, Stevens MB, Shulman LE (1979) The "C.R.E.S.T." syndrome — comparison with systemic sclerosis (scleroderma). Arch Intern Med 139: 1240–1244

Zeek PM (1953) Periarteritis nodosa and other forms of necrotising angiitis. N Engl J Med 148: 764–768

13 The General Principles of Management of Chronic Arthritis in the Context of a Patient with Rheumatoid Arthritis

Introduction

The bland statement "there is nothing more to be done" is frequently made to the patient with chronic arthritis and reflects observer ignorance and indifference. There is much palliative, supportive and reconstructive care which can and should be provided at each stage in the disease. If a medical practitioner feels unable to offer constructive aid, consultation with medical and paramedical colleagues is mandatory. There is always something which can be done, and a disabled patient who is looking for help should not be disappointed. The following points are relevant (and should be read in conjunction with relevant sections in Chaps. 2, 3 and 4).

Assess, Discuss, Educate, Reassess

Full medical and social assessment is the first step in management. Thereafter discussion with the patient and family or friends is important. The choice of treatment should reflect both the severity of the disease and the expectations of the patient. Some uncertainty in predicting the course of disease and likely response to therapy is inevitable, and the medical practitioner needs to show cautious optimism tempered with realism. The constant aim is to minimise disability, but denial of disease makes achievement of this aim more difficult. Above all, throughout all management of such patients must run strongly the thread of constantly defining and refining the therapeutic goals and of monitoring the progress of the patient towards the achievement of these goals.

Multidisciplinary Teams

Heroic pharmacological or surgical measures are rarely necessary: many of the skills of the multi-disciplinary team will be neglected if the medical practitioner sees no further than multi-coloured capsules and prosthetic joints. "Shared care" is not merely a catch phrase but is essential in the management of chronic arthritis. Members of this team include:

1. Patient
2. Family and extended family
3. Employer/religious advisor
4. Community organisers (housing, transport, welfare, disablement resettlement officer, voluntary organisations, e.g. arthritis care, disabled incomes group etc.)
5. Paramedical staff (hospital and community): nurse, physiotherapist, occupational therapist, medical social worker, chiropodist, pharmacist, orthotist
6. Medical practitioners: general, medical and surgical

Co-ordination in the team requires careful planning and frequent reassessment. Leadership is important since the patient needs to feel that someone is in command of the situation and a coherent plan needs to be followed by all. The leader of the team will vary according to circumstances but is usually the general or hospital practitioner. Some autocracy may be necessary to ensure that one aspect is not unduly emphasised at the expense of others. Case conferences which allow group discussion of individual problems are helpful.

General Measures

These are of considerable importance and should provide a background for drug and surgical treatment.

Rest and Exercise

Many patients ask about the advisability of exercise and the importance of striking a balance between rest and exercise should be stressed. The majority learn to adjust their lifestyle to variations in activity of their disease, and no active intervention is required. Acute inflammation may necessitate splinting or bed rest or a combination of the two. As the acute phase settles, gradual mobilisation should begin. Frequent gentle exercise is almost invariably preferable to occasional major exertion. Patients should be cautioned never to push themselves to the point of exhaustion. Specific exercises are indicated to strengthen muscles, e.g. quadriceps, or to aid post-operative mobilisation which should be supervised by the physiotherapist.

Splints

Splinting should achieve two broad goals. Firstly splints should rest acutely inflamed joints in a position of optimum function and give symptomatic relief. Secondly serial splinting should correct postural deformity and partly restore function. Wrist splints both working and resting and serial knee splints are most frequently used, and many joints may be improved by this relatively simple method. Hip traction will have an effect similar to splinting of other joints but should only be used in the short term.

Cervical Collars

Cervical collars also play a dual role. They will act symptomatically as a splint where active disease of the cervical spine is producing pain, and protectively where destructive disease endangers neurological function. There has been recent controversy about the latter role, but in general a firm collar is advised to give protection to the spinal cord in atlanto-axial instability and should always be worn when unexpected positional change is likely. A soft collar will give symptomatic relief and is particularly recommended for night time use. Any evidence of neurological impairment requires prompt surgical assessment. Habitual use of a collar in mild disease is best discouraged since it fosters dependency and distracts from the more important long-term goal of mobilisation, activity and regular exercises.

Footwear

The need for suitable footwear seems self-evident but is often ignored. Vanity, difficulty in getting out to shop or poverty may be relevant and all should be considered and dealt with appropriately. Simple measures such as metatarsal pads correctly worn may give sustained relief to the rheumatoid patient. The chiropodist and specialist shoemaker can contribute much to foot care. The availability of more appropriate lighter plastics has been a considerable advance in this area.

Aids

The physiotherapist, occupational therapist and social services alone or together can transform the lives of disabled patients by the provision of simple, or occasionally more sophisticated aids. Every moderately or severely affected patient deserves access to their skills: assessment and reassessment over the years is required. A walking stick used in the wrong hand, or one inherited from a stunted rachitic grandfather and consequently too short, is an unnecessary handicap. Eating, drinking, washing, toileting and dressing are fundamental daily activities where lack of independence causes embarrass-ment and depression, yet where even minor improvements will boost morale. Very often the best functional aid for a patient and the one most likely to be used is the one which they design for themselves.

Social Support, Literature

A combined approach by social workers, disablement resettlement officers and housing managers is required to provide as suitable an environment as possible. If the patient agrees, discussion with employers or family may allow continuation of work, even if hours or type of occupation requires adjustment, or special adaptations are necessary. The present disastrous economic climate adds to the burden of these chronically disabled patients and it becomes even more important that the physician attempts everything in his power to avert the threat of redundancy. Once out of work it is common to observe disease deterioration.

A supply of informative literature (notably from the ARC), tailored where possible to individual needs, should be made available to the patient and complement formal consultations.

Philosophy of Approach to Drug Therapy

An outline of a scheme for drug therapy in chronic arthritis is shown in Table 13.1. Drugs are grouped into three broad categories, viz. first, second and third line. Most patients with osteoarthritis or inflammatory disease will require first line drugs if only at one or other stage during the course of their disease. It is only in patients with rheumatoid arthritis that consideration of possible institution of second or third line drugs may be appropriate, and even then only in a minority of these patients. It must be emphasised that second line drugs have no place in the management of patients with osteoarthritis.

First Line Drugs

First line non-steroidal anti-inflammatory drugs (NSAID) diminish pain and stiffness but do not exert an effect on the underlying disease process. The majority of rheumatoid patients need this type of medication every day, and all

Table 13.1. Scheme of drug therapy in patients with rheumatoid arthritis

First line	Non-steroidal antirheumatic drugs
	Choose on the basis of patient preference
	Select the single best compromise between efficacy and lack of side-effects
	Dose varied to suit the needs of the time
	Do not affect the underlying disease
Second line	Gold
	Penicillamine
	Antimalarials
	Others, e.g. levamisole
	Potentially extremely toxic
	Must be monitored meticulously
	May influence the underlying disease
Third line	Cytotoxic drugs
	Corticosteroids/? ACTH
	Under most unusual circumstances
	Plasmaphoresis
	Irradiation
	Leucophoresis

possible measures to increase drug efficacy and to minimise toxicity should be employed. A large number of these drugs have recently become available. The question of which drug to use is difficult and there is no simple answer. In the first instance, however, there are broad principles which should be followed:

1. Become familiar with five or six NSAIDs. Know the dose, preparations, anticipated efficacy and possible side-effects of each. It is preferable to prescribe the better established older drugs rather than to ring the changes with the most recently introduced, most powerfully marketed "Mac brufens".

2. Use one drug at a time, up to full dosage, and encourage patients who complain of lack of effect to persevere for 2 weeks before abandoning that drug.

3. Ensure that patient expectation is realistic. These drugs will not abolish pain completely, although they should produce considerable symptomatic relief when properly used.

4. Instruct patients to vary the dose according to their symptoms. Compliance is not a problem here—a drug which produces pain relief without unacceptable side-effects will be taken. Patients soon learn what they require and will adjust their own treatment satisfactorily. Admittedly some will exceed the suggested maximum or add their own combinations of patent medicines, and a detailed history must be taken without hostility.

5. Be certain of previous therapy. Many patients do not consider aspirin a drug since they can self prescribe. The pharmaceutical companies have shown consideration in at least producing different colours and shapes of capsules and tablets, and an identification card is often of help in elucidating the problem. We have a plastic display folder containing labelled samples of the drugs in the clinic and find this most valuable. It is good practice and helpful to all concerned for the patient to be provided with a drug card upon which all

medications which he or she is receiving may be recorded. All patients should know what drugs they are taking and why.

6. Pay attention to dispensing methods. Childproof containers or even ordinary bottles pose a problem for the arthritic patient. Similarly, suppositories may be impracticable in some circumstances.

7. Vary the timing of therapy according to symptoms. If morning stiffness is a major problem a large bedtime dose may prove to be effective. Drugs with prolonged half-lives which are taken once a day do not always allow this flexibility but may be useful for those with mild disease who find a single daily dose more convenient. It should not need to be stated that "morning stiffness" in a night-shift worker becomes evening stiffness.

Bearing in mind these general principles, the next step is to select the optimum single first line drug. This is based upon patient preference. It is worthwhile offering the patient a series of five or six first line drugs, being guided by the familiarity of the physician with the drugs concerned. Each drug should be taken for at least 7 days commencing in low or middling dose but making sure to end each period at the highest permissible dose. The patient records at the end of each week on a 0 to 10 scale efficacy and any adverse effects encountered. It is most unusual to find a patient who cannot opt for a single best drug in this way. It is important to emphasise to the patient that these drugs may reduce but will not abolish pain and stiffness altogether. Rather the aim of treatment is to select the drug which relieves the symptoms best without producing side-effects. Thereafter the patient should take that preferred drug in the minimum dose tailored to suit the needs of his or her symptoms, discontinuing completely during periods of remission. Unfortunately there is no method that predicts which patient will respond to which drug.

General Points About Individual Drugs

In very active disease, and especially in young patients, indomethacin is a useful drug. The dose may range as high as 250 or even 300 mg per day. High dose aspirin is also useful in some patients in these same circumstances but again the high dose cannot be prescribed on a sustained basis. Ibuprofen is perhaps less powerful but has the conspicuous advantage of being well tolerated and may be tried first in those with mild disease. There is no longer a role for phenylbutazone or oxyphenbutazone in rheumatoid arthritis. If a drug is effective and non-toxic the number of capsules or tablets required and the timing of these are of little consequence. When dysphagia is present, a suspension such as benorylate (or indomethacin or naproxen) may be invaluable.

Special Circumstances

Gastrointestinal Side-effects

No effective anti-inflammatory agent is free of gastrointestinal side-effects, but a change of preparation, or timing or route of administration may alleviate symptoms. If dyspepsia persists, investigation and where necessary appropriate management of peptic ulcer should be undertaken. Surgeons and gastroenterologists usually recommend cessation of anti-inflammatory drugs, but this is virtually impossible in some patients with active inflammatory joint disease. The minimum dose of NSAID should be tried and in patients with rheumatoid arthritis second line drugs may be considered somewhat earlier than usual; nevertheless, the gastrointestinal problem will often need to be managed against a background of anti-inflammatory medication.

Diarrhoea occurs most commonly with the fenamates, especially in older patients, and discontinuation of therapy is usually required. Indomethacin should be avoided in the elderly, if only because of its propensity to produce fluid retention.

Analgesics

Analgesics have little or no effect in active inflammatory disease but do have a role in post-operative care and in patients with advanced destructive disease with little inflammation. Opiates are never indicated for more than the immediate postoperative period—not only are they unhelpful but addiction is a real risk.

Very severe pain requires investigation and treatment of causes such as infection or fracture. When these have been excluded, appropriate rest for the affected joint and either vigorous anti-inflammatory therapy or surgery may be indicated. In certain circumstances we have found that assistance from our local pain relief clinic has been invaluable.

Interaction with Other Drugs

1. *Anticoagulants*. Many anti-inflammatory drugs do interact with warfarin, but ibuprofen, flurbiprofen, indomethacin and tolmetin may be used in patients where anticoagulation is mandatory. Be alert for gastrointestinal complications of the NSAID.

2. *Oral hypoglycaemics*. Feprazone, naproxen and sulindac are contraindicated.

3. *Antihypertensives and diuretics*. Interactions with indomethacin and piroxicam have been observed and it is wise to avoid concurrent prescription. The same may well prove to be the case with all other prostaglandin synthetase inhibitors since this is the probable mechanism of production of this effect.

Pregnancy

While many rheumatoid arthritis patients improve during pregnancy, a few will still require anti-inflammatory drugs. Salicylates are the drug of choice and the dose should be as low as possible. In the last trimester the situation should be revised since anti-inflammatory doses of salicylates may prolong gestation and possibly increase the incidence of stillbirth. There is no firm evidence of a teratogenic effect when salicylate is used during the first trimester. Indomethacin has been reported to cause premature closure of the ductus arteriosus and should be avoided in pregnancy.

Failure of First Line Drugs (N.B. Only applicable to patients with rheumatoid arthritis)

Where active disease persists despite optimum use of non-steroidal anti-inflammatory drugs and general supportive measures, reassessment of local disease, generalised disease and the patient's circumstances is necessary. If disease is local, (a) ensure that no infection is present and that the diagnosis is correct and (b) consider intensive physiotherapy, intra-articular aspiration, lavage and instillation of corticosteroid, and possibly surgical opinion. If disease is generalised, (a) ensure that there is no other reason for deterioration, that all options have been explored and that full assessment has been completed and (b) consider a short spell in hospital and use of second line drugs.

It is important to recognise that patient dissatisfaction alone is insufficient reason to proceed to more vigorous treatment. Subjective complaints without objective evidence of inflammation and destruction suggest that patient expectation is unrealistic or that problems other than rheumatoid arthritis must be considered. A careful reappraisal is thus necessary before embarking on more hazardous therapy. In addition, complications of the disease and co-diseases must be dealt with (Chap. 8).

On the opposite extreme some patients who have progressive disease poorly controlled by first line drugs are reluctant to co-operate with more intensive therapy. In this situation comprehensive explanation of therapeutic goals and regular review are indicated. There is never a justification to bully or even cajole a patient against her or his wishes. Second line drugs are toxic preparations and while rheumatoid arthritis may be a severe disabling disease it is rarely in itself life threatening.

Second Line Drugs

Second line drugs are indicated for the minority of patients with rheumatoid arthritis who have progressive generalised disease which is not controlled after an unhurried trial of the measures discussed above. There is some evidence that in responding patients these drugs may influence the course of the disease favourably. They will not relieve pain directly, nor alter established deformity. Clearly however, if inflammatory activity is reduced, there will be gradual relief of pain. In addition, deformity may be preventable but this has not yet been proven. When continued for 18 months or more there is some evidence that drugs in this category will slow the rate of appearance of erosions, a crucial point which requires further controlled study over prolonged periods.

However, the need to withhold second line drugs from patients with active disease for 2 years or more makes such controlled studies very difficult. Leaving aside the question of radiological improvement, systemic features of rheumatoid arthritis such as lethargy, weight loss and anaemia may show improvement during successful second line therapy.

In view of the potential toxic effects of these compounds, patient co-operation is mandatory. Maximal benefit is delayed for 6 weeks or even several months, and patients accustomed to the almost immediate symptomatic benefit of first line drugs need to understand the therapeutic goal. They also need support so that they will persevere with therapy. The concept of continuing first line therapy in parallel needs explanation, especially when patients have been used to a routine of "one drug at a time" and varying the dose themselves to suit the needs of their symptoms at the time. There is *no* place for such patient participation in the management of second line drugs.

The lack of initial improvement means that patient compliance cannot automatically be assumed. Toxic effects are of a different nature from those of first line drugs and are often not apparent to the patient. While limited patient education should facilitate sensible use of first line drugs with minimal intervention, there is no substitute for constant medical supervision of second line therapy. The practice of "covering" the institution of second line drugs with corticosteroids is to be deprecated. Only a minority of patients commenced on, for example, gold will respond well without side-effects, leaving the majority at risk of continuing requirement for long-term low dose corticosteroid therapy: a disastrous outcome. Three to four months is not long in the context of the patient's disease history, which might well extend for up to 40 or 50 years. Lastly the additional complexity of assessing the patient starting simultaneously both gold and prednisolone should give the physician cause for thought.

Contenders for the description "second line" drugs are gold, penicillamine, antimalarial agents and possibly others, such as levamisole. Again, the question arises—which drug? In part the answer will depend on the experience and interest of the medical practitioner and the facilities available for monitoring. Gold and penicillamine are the best established second line drugs and in terms of overall efficacy and toxicity there is little to choose between them.

Conditions required before embarking on either drug are:

1. Cooperative, informed, reliable patient and family
2. Realistic therapeutic goal and methods to assess the response towards that goal
3. Conscientious medical practitioner and locum
4. Facilities to check urine, blood and skin at each visit
5. Normal white cell and differential count and platelets
6. Normal urine, blood urea and electrolytes

A monitoring card which documents drug dose, urinalysis and blood results at each visit is essential and diminishes the potential for error.

The influence of previous second line therapy on the subsequent efficacy or development of toxicity on another is relevant since many patients will be treated with more than one of these drugs over the course of their disease. Results have been conflicting but we have not been able to show any adverse effect of prior gold on subsequent penicillamine therapy or vice versa.

Intramuscular gold ensures compliance since monitoring at the time of injection can always be carried out. Both drugs require frequent early monitoring but in the long term 4-weekly visits are sufficient. Drop out rates because of toxicity are high (30%–40% in the first year) and if disease activity persists or recurs the alternative drug may be tried. The interval between the two therapies does not appear to influence subsequent toxicity in our studies, nevertheless a period of 3 months between cessation of one drug and commencement of a second allows toxic effects to reverse (and obviously they should have disappeared altogether before another drug is contemplated) and also allows reassessment of disease activity. In some instances benefit derived from a second line drug will last for many months after toxicity has necessitated withdrawal of therapy.

Third Line Drugs

Treatments under this heading are used only when other measures have failed, despite conscientious efforts on all sides. Some therapies in this category are experimental and their role may change as more evidence about efficacy and toxicity becomes available.

Azathioprine and Cyclophosphamide

These two drugs have both been shown to exert an effect in rheumatoid arthritis in that over a period of months indices of activity will diminish in responding patients and the rate of radiological progression may be slower. As indicated in Chap. 17, however, doubts about toxicity, especially in the long-term, limit their use in a disease such as rheumatoid arthritis, which is usually not fatal. Azathioprine is the less toxic of the two and should probably be tried first. Some patients will recognise the drugs (or side-effects such as alopecia) as those associated with therapy for malignancy and careful explanation is necessary. Neither of these drugs is recommended in younger age groups.

Corticosteroids

As discussed in Chap. 18, corticosteroids have a very limited role in rheumatoid arthritis. It is important to recognise that their use involves not an abdication of responsibility but rather a commitment to close monitoring and constant attempts to minimise toxicity. This, of course, is true of many of the toxic compounds employed in rheumatology, but is stressed here since the prompt initial sense of well-being experienced by the patient may produce a false sense of security. Every clinician who starts therapy should try to envisage managing the same patient 10 or 20 years later, with iatrogenic disease superimposed on the original complaint. Systemic steroids should never be used in an unreliable patient who may abuse the dose regimen. These reservations apply less to topical or intra-articular steroid, which if correctly used should have minimal systemic toxicity.

Plasmapheresis, Lymphatic Drainage and Nodal Irradiation

These procedures are experimental and require further study before their role, if any, is elucidated.

Alternative Medicine

It is not surprising that many patients resort to alternative medicine at some stage of their disease. It should be stressed, however, that there is no scientific evidence of efficacy of diet, copper bangle, herbal remedies, acupuncture etc., and if they are to be tried it is important that toxicity should not result. Disposable needles should be used by the acupuncturist, and idiosyncratic reactions to herbal remedies should be borne in mind. In addition the financial burden of this type of treatment may be considerable and may stress the limited resourses of the disabled patient and family.

Further Reading

Gerber LH (1981) Principles and their application in the rehabilitation of patients with rheumatic disease. In: Kelly W, Harris ED Jr, Ruddy S, Sledge CB (eds) Textbook of rheumatology, 1st edn. Saunders, Philadelphia London Toronto, Chap 112
Hill AGS (1978) General management of rheumatoid arthritis. In: Scott JT (ed) Copeman's textbook of the rheumatic diseases, 5th edn. Churchill Livingstone, Edinburgh London New York, pp 391–403
Ruddy S (1981) The management of rheumatoid arthritis. In: Kelly W, Harris ED Jr, Ruddy S, Sledge CB (eds) Textbook of rheumatology, 1st edn. Saunders, Philadelphia London Toronto, Chap 63

14 Pharmacology of the Drugs Used in the Treatment of Chronic Arthritis

Introduction

This section is devoted to description of the drugs used in this field beyond the context of individual diseases. Apart from certain unusual instances such as the deployment of the appropriate antibiotic in a patient with infectious arthritis or the prescription of allopurinol in gout, most of rheumatology consists of the management of patients with chronic incurable disease on a symptomatic basis. The drugs prescribed do not exert a specific effect upon the pathological basis of the disease but rather are prescribed to relieve symptoms and thereby hopefully to improve function and the patient's ability to cope with the presence of the disease. Much of this concept has been stressed beforehand in the context of the individual diseases. It is on this basis that the doctrine of *primum non nocere* becomes central.

All of the drugs discussed in this chapter are first line antirheumatic drugs (Table 14.1)

Aspirin

The healing properties of the willow bark have been recognised for centuries, the discovery probably owing a great deal to the goddess of advances in medicine, serendipity.

Aspirin (acetylsalicylic acid) is administered orally, maximum absorption occurring at pH 2.5–4.0. The rate and completeness of absorption is influenced by a wide variety of factors, including particle size and formulation, gastric motility and blood flow and rate of dissolution of the preparation prescribed. In the stomach aspirin may interfere with the "back diffusion" of hydrogen ions.

Table 14.1. First line antirheumatic drugs[a]

Salicylates (and related compounds)	Aspirin (acetylsalycylic acid), Levius, Safapryn, Nuseal, Benoral, aloxiprin, Salsalate, Paynocil, diflunisal, trisilate
Propionic acids derivatives	Ibuprofen, ketoprofen, fenoprofen, naproxen, flurbiprofen, tiaprofenic acid, fenbufen, indoprofen
Phenylacetic acids	Diclofenac, fenclofenac
Indoleacetic acids	Indomethacin, tolmetin
Indene derivatives	Sulindac
Fenamates	Mefenamic acid, flufenamic acid
Oxicam derivatives	Piroxicam
Benzotriazine	Azapropazone
Pyrazole derivatives	Feprazone

[a] Phenylbutazone and oxyphenylbutazone belong here chemically but should be counted clinically as second line drugs

After absorption aspirin is transported bound to albumin. The degree and the strength of binding of aspirin in relationship to other drugs and indeed to endogenous substances is important. The more highly and tightly bound the molecule, the less likely it is to be displaced. The consequences of displacement can easily be predicted with a thorough knowledge of the pharmacology of the compounds concerned. Displacement will release free drug, which will then be metabolised and excreted more rapidly. This will often lead to a reduction in efficacy and adverse reactions associated with the displaced drug. In some situations, however, the drug (or the pro-drug) in itself is ineffective and the effect is produced by metabolism to active molecules. In this case displacement may result in enhancement of efficacy and of adverse reactions. Again, metabolism may yield either a compound which is effective without the side-effects of the parent compound or a compound which is ineffective but produces adverse reactions that are distinct from those of the parent compound. It is also worth being aware of the mathematics of displacement. One per cent displacement of a drug which is 100% tightly protein bound will produce a 10% increase in the concentration of free drug.

Aspirin is metabolised in the hepatocyte by a variety of different routes. Some of these metabolic pathways display saturable kinetics with the result that a small increase in administered dose may produce a disproportionate rise in serum salicylate concentrations. This is the explanation for the narrow therapeutic ratio of high dose treatment.

Serum concentrations on regular dosing rise to a plateau towards the end of 1 week but in some individuals there may be a continuing slow increase lasting for several weeks. Synovial fluid concentrations equilibrate at about half of the serum concentration. Excretion occurs through the kidney. Only a small proportion of the ingested dose appears as aspirin, the remainder as metabolites.

Adverse Reactions

Gastrointestinal

Aspirin produces a wide range of metabolic and endocrine effects in addition to the desired anti-inflammatory action. These include expansion of the plasma volume, complex effects in different doses upon acid-base balance, hypoglycaemia and increased metabolic rate due to uncoupling of oxidative phosphorylation.

The most significant effect from the point of view of the physician is upon the gastrointestinal tract, where dyspepsia and bleeding are common. The incidence of dyspepsia ranges from 10% to 50% in different studies and is dose related.

The basis of these toxic effects on the gastric mucosa is not yet clear and it may well be that other factors such as alcohol, minor degrees of coagulopathy or hypovitaminosis C may contribute. At least part of the effect is local and blood loss is unrelated to dyspepsia. Bleeding is a function of the acetyl group since it is much less pronounced with salicylic acid itself.

It is probable that some individuals will develop frank haemorrhage from the gastrointestinal tract when exposed to aspirin. This is a rare event in the context of the enormous numbers of patients who have been exposed to high doses of aspirin over many years and is probably idiosyncratic. Again, there is no relationship between those who develop major haemorrhage and those who suffer dyspepsia or minor bleeding and the other factors mentioned above may exert an additive effect. There are now so many safer alternatives that it is not justified to re-expose a patient who has suffered this complication, but this has been done in the past and those who bled the first time do not necessarily do so again on re-exposure.

Similarly, it is likely that aspirin does play a role in the production of gastric if not duodenal peptic ulceration but it is probable that this represents one factor in a multivariate analysis, others being of equal or greater importance. There is no doubt that aspirin may produce acute gastric erosions.

In the liver, aspirin will produce acute liver cell damage in children and in some adults at the onset of treatment with high doses. The evidence that aspirin will produce chronic liver disease is lacking, even when it is given in large doses over many years, and again it is possible that this effect may be idiosyncratic and time locked.

Haematological

Aspirin will produce major effects on coagulation and platelets in very low doses. This is a function of the acetyl group and depends upon the irreversible acetylation of red cell and platelet membrane protein. Thus once exposed to even 300 mg aspirin in a single dose these structures will be abnormal for the rest of their existence and tests reflecting this effect will remain abnormal until a new non-acetylated population has replaced them. Bleeding time is prolonged and coagulation tests are disturbed, making it important to record details of aspirin ingestion. In a very few patients aspirin may cause reversible pancytopenia, and aspirin may produce haemolysis in patients with glucose-6-phosphatase deficiency.

Renal

In a manner analogous to the acute effect on the hepatocyte, aspirin produces a rise in the urinary cell count at the commencement of treatment and the effect of aspirin may be monitored by a reduction in creatinine clearance and a rise in the concentration in urine of an enzyme which reflects very sensitively renal tubular cell function (NAG or N-acetyl glucosamine). At least part of the effect of aspirin on the kidney may be mediated by aspirin-induced changes in prostaglandin-controlled renal blood flow. Evidence that aspirin produces chronic renal impairment is lacking.

Hypersensitivity

Aspirin hypersensitivity is very rare indeed but may present as a skin rash, urticaria and angioneurotic oedema or asthma. Patients with a family history of allergy, nasal polyps or eczema are at risk and such individuals may exhibit "allergy" to a wide array of chemical compounds and drugs. A patient with aspirin allergy is liable to develop a similar adverse reaction with many of the other first line drugs. It has been suggested that the mechanism depends upon the prostaglandin system and is not a true specific IgE-mediated allergy. It is worth ascertaining whether or not such patients also suffer from Sjögren's syndrome.

Interactions

Interactions between aspirin and other drugs are frequent yet rarely lead to overt clinical problems if the philosophy of management advocated in this book is followed. These may occur before, during or after absorption, during transport or intermediary metabolism and at the level of excretion. As always, the way to be certain of avoiding interactions is to prescribe drugs singly whenever possible and to be alert for potential interactions by being aware of the pharmacology of the drugs concerned where this is not possible.

   The other side-effect of aspirin which is well known to all patients who have taken this drug in high dose is ototoxicity. This may be manifest as tinnitus or sometimes as the insidious development of deafness without any associated symptoms. It is important to be aware of this side-effect, which shows wide variation in individual threshold.

Prescription

Aspirin is best prescribed as soluble aspirin in 300 mg tablets. It has been shown that high doses (>3.6 g/day) are required to produce an anti-inflammatory effect as measured by reduction in finger joint swelling but it has never been established that such high doses are required on a continuing basis. Whatever the truth of this, one thing is certain: Very few patients will continue to take such high doses over prolonged periods. It is possible that we are in danger of discarding an effective remedy because of incorrect prescribing practices. Some patients (10–15%) with rheumatoid arthritis choose aspirin as their preferred drug and continue to take this in variable dose tailored to suit the needs of their own symptoms quite happily for many years. Conspicuously, these patients maintain their dose below that required to produce side-effects and this may be the best way to prescribe aspirin in the chronic rheumatic diseases. It is also noteworthy that such patients select their own formulation and adjust frequency and mode of administration to suit their own needs.

If an adverse reaction is encountered at a dose too low to produce efficacy then it is important to change to another drug and not to persevere with aspirin to the patient's detriment. If dyspepsia is encountered in a patient who is responding well, then it is sometimes worth prescribing aspirin to be taken after meals (which retard and reduce the absorption peak but do not reduce total bioavailability) or an antacid. It is best to avoid those which contain bicarbonate or aluminium. Bicarbonate has a complex effect upon bioavailability, and aluminium may complex with aspirin in the gut.

Indomethacin

Indomethacin has been used widely throughout the world for over 15 years in the treatment of chronic rheumatic diseases and has found a new role in the laboratory as the prototype inhibitor of prostaglandin synthetases. It is an indoleacetic acid derivative [1-(p-chlorobenzoyl)-5-methoxy-2-methylindole-acetic acid], insoluble in water but soluble in alcohol, and must be protected from direct sunlight.

It is well absorbed following oral administration, peak serum concentrations occurring within $\frac{1}{2}$ to 2 h after ingestion, and pain relief follows closely the graph of serum concentration against time. At a later stage pain relief persists beyond the time when the serum concentration has dropped to unmeasurable values and it is suggested that there is a "deep pool" in peripheral tissues where the metabolites are recycled into active drug.

Indomethacin is metabolised in the hepatocyte by O-demethylation and N-deacylation and there is an enterohepatic recirculation. Approximately 66% of the dose ingested is excreted in the urine as the glucuronide and 30% is excreted in the faeces unchanged. The concentration in synovial fluid rises more slowly than serum initially but later it exceeds it. Indomethacin is absorbed equally well from the rectum and recently a "slow release" oral formulation has been introduced.

Indomethacin is a highly effective anti-inflammatory agent which is best prescribed alone and is especially effective in the treatment of rheumatoid arthritis, gout and ankylosing spondylitis. It will provide relief of symptoms in non-articular rheumatism, osteoarthritis and degenerative disc disease but many safer alternatives are available and should be tried first. A great deal of emphasis has been placed upon the practice of prescribing a large dose of indomethacin late at night in order to relieve morning stiffness and this is undoubtedly effective. It is also good prescribing practice to treat the primary symptom, i.e. pain at night, which may prevent the patient from getting to sleep. It is more sensible to treat the pain than to prescribe a hypnotic, which may in fact make the symptoms worse. On the other hand it is likely that the same effect may be obtained by providing late at night a large dose of whichever NSAID drug the patient is receiving during the day in exactly the same way.

Indomethacin may be prescribed in different ways. In a fit young male who has developed a highly inflammatory disease such as acute gout or active severe ankylosing spondylitis, it is reasonable to commence with a very high dose and reduce in proportion to relief of symptoms. In an elderly frail patient with a less inflammatory process such as osteoarthritis, a different drug would probably be preferred; however, if for some reason indomethacin was chosen, then treatment would commence with a much lower dose (25 mg t.i.d.) or the equivalent and increase only gradually to the lowest dose which will provide relief without producing side-effects. It is in these circumstances that the addition of a large dose, taken as the patient is already settled in bed ready to go to sleep, will provide prolonged relief of symptoms lasting into the morning. The theory is that any minor side-effects occur while the patient is asleep.

Tolmetin (Tolectin; 1-methyl-5-*p*-toluoylpyrrole-2-acetic acid)

Tolmetin is a pyrrole with structural similarities to indomethacin. Like indomethacin, it is a prostaglandin synthetase inhibitor and shows antipyretic, analgesic and anti-inflammatory activity in animal models. It interferes with platelet function and prolongs the bleeding time, although this is not clinically significant.

Absorption is complete after oral administration, peak plasma concentrations appearing within 30–40 min, and absorption is not reduced by antacids. It has a plasma half-life of 4.5–6.0 h and the volume of distribution is about 9 litres. The drug is highly (99%) protein bound and most of the ingested dose is excreted within 24 h, 70% as the dicarboxylic metabolite. There is no evidence of accumulation and metabolism does not change with prolonged administration. Concurrent aspirin treatment will reduce the serum concentration of tolmetin but the converse does not apply. Gastrointestinal blood loss is less than with aspirin or indomethacin and tolmetin produces less central nervous system side-effects than indomethacin. However, dyspepsia is still troublesome in approximately one-quarter of patients, and nausea, vomiting and even upper abdominal pain will be encountered. Other adverse reactions include tinnitus, fluid retention oedema and elevation of blood pressure and skin rash.

Tolmetin sodium is prescribed as 200 mg (or 400 mg double strength) tablets three or four times per day; smaller doses may be adequate in the elderly or in osteoarthritis.

The Propionic Acid Derivatives

Ibuprofen

The propionic acid series of compounds was discovered in 1960 by the Boots company in England. Drugs from this series are now the drugs of first choice in the chronic inflammatory and degenerative joint diseases. This has occurred not so much on the basis of improved efficacy but rather because these compounds produce less frequent and less severe adverse reactions than their competitors.

Ibuprofen [2-(4-isobutylphenyl) propionic acid] is a prostaglandin synthetase inhibitor which has anti-inflammatory, analgesic and antipyretic activity in animal and in man. It stabilises lysosomal and other membranes, inhibits Trafuril erythema, uncouples oxidative phosphorylation and inhibits histamine release. It has no effect upon the cardiovascular, respiratory or central nervous systems, nor upon corticosteroid or other hormone production as far as has been determined to date. Recent data on the general effects of all drugs of this class does raise the suspicion that there may be effects upon renal blood supply and possibly upon calcium metabolism, and this field needs to be followed closely.

Ibuprofen is rapidly absorbed following oral administration and peak blood levels are attained within 2–3 h. When it is taken before meals, absorption is delayed and peak blood concentrations are reduced. It has a short half-life (2–4 h), is only loosely protein bound and is metabolised in the hepatocyte to two inert metabolites. It does not affect mixed oxidases in the liver. All of the administered dose is excreted in the urine in the form of the metabolites within 24 h and there is no accumulation. With continuous administration, equilibrium is reached within 5–7 days.

Ibuprofen is a remarkably safe drug, the only significant side-effect being dyspepsia, which is rarely severe. The dose varies widely between 1 and 3 g per day in divided doses according to circumstances. There is no interference with anticoagulation or antidepressant regimens.

Thus ibuprofen is a very safe antirheumatic drug although it may be less effective than aspirin or indomethacin. Few problems of drug interactions are encountered with ibuprofen. It is ideal for many patients with non-articular rheumatism, degenerative arthritis or early and mild cases of inflammatory arthritis.

Fenoprofen Calcium

This is a calcium salt of [*d,l*,-2-(3-phenoxyphenyl)propionic acid] which is a white crystalline powder only slightly soluble in water but highly soluble in 95% alcohol. It has a pH of between 4 and 5, which favours rapid absorption from the stomach, and exists as a racemic mixture, both the D and the L isomers being equally active.

Fenoprofen is an effective anti-inflammatory, analgesic and antipyretic compound which has a similar range of in vitro activities to the other propionic acid drugs. After oral administration it is rapidly absorbed and transported bound to plasma albumin. The binding constant is high; thus fenoprofen will tend to displace other less tightly bound molecules. Metabolic products, particularly the glucuronides, are formed in the liver. These are transported to and excreted in the kidney. The route of elimination is predominantly renal, so care should be exercised in the presence of renal failure. Peak plasma concentrations occur within 60 min of oral administration. Food delays absorption and concurrent aspirin administration reduces the peak plasma concentration. This effect is bidirectional.

Fenoprofen is an effective antirheumatic in the treatment of rheumatoid arthritis, osteoarthritis, and the seronegative spondarthritides and produces greater analgesia in non-articular syndromes than do simple analgesics. Adverse reactions are those familiar from the other members of this group of drugs and may exhibit a degree of individualism in their manifestation. Dyspepsia is the most commonly encountered adverse reaction and skin rashes are rare.

The dose range lies between 600 mg and 2.4 g, and the amount taken should be the minimum required to achieve the therapeutic goal. This will vary widely according to the age, weight and sex of the patient and the disease being treated and is best selected by the patient. Fenoprofen is available in 300 and 600 mg tablets and as 300 mg water dispensable tablets (Fenopron D). Onset of action begins promptly within 60 min of administration, but maximum effect may be delayed for 1–2 weeks of regular administration.

Ketoprofen

Ketoprofen is 2-(3-benzoylphenyl) propionic acid, which is a white crystalline powder. Its mode of action and spectrum of adverse reactions are similar to those of the other members of this group of drugs, as are its properties in vitro and in animal models.

Ketoprofen is rapidly absorbed, peak concentrations in plasma occurring within 30 min after intramuscular, 60 min after rectal and 90 min after oral administration. The corresponding biological half-lives are approximately 1 h, 2 h and 2 h respectively. These figures apply to single doses and a plateau is reached after 48–96 h of regular administration without any subsequent evidence of accumulation. Ketoprofen circulates loosely bound to plasma proteins, mainly albumin, and is metabolised in the hepatocyte and excreted through the renal tubular cells. Synovial fluid concentrations rise slowly to meet those of paired serum samples and may even exceed them.

Attempts have been made to derive tables of equivalent potency to compare ketoprofen with the other first line drugs but these are somewhat specious. There is greater variability between different patients in this respect than between different drugs.

Ketoprofen is an effective antirheumatic drug in a wide array of arthritides and is well tolerated. The most common adverse reaction encountered after oral administration is dyspepsia. "Allergy" may occur with this as with most of the other first line drugs but this is very rare. Ketoprofen is available as 50 or 100 mg tablets and as a 50 mg suppository. The dose varies widely between 100 mg and 200 mg in accordance with patient preference. A new sustained release capsule is available.

Naproxen

Naproxen [2-(6-methoxy-2-naphthyl)propionic acid] is an odourless crystalline powder which is active as the d-isomer. It is highly lipid soluble but is only water soluble at physiological pH. Its spectrum of activity in vitro in animal models and in vivo in man is similar to the other members of this group. It inhibits the second phase of platelet aggregation and may thus prolong the bleeding time.

Naproxen is well absorbed after oral administration, peak plasma levels occurring 1–2 h after ingestion. Antacids or food retard and reduce absorption. It is transported tightly bound to plasma proteins, from which it will displace other protein-bound drugs such as warfarin, sulphonylureas, hydantoins and probenecid, and has a prolonged half-life (12–14 h) which permits dosage on a b.d. basis. Concurrent treatment with aspirin will reduce the plasma concentration. Drug clearance increases as plasma concentration increases and accumulation does not occur. Naproxen is conjugated in the hepatocyte with glucuronide and is also demethylated. It crosses the placenta and is secreted in breast milk, as are all the other drugs of this class. Approximately 95% is excreted in the urine, 10% free and the rest as the glucuronidated or demethylated metabolite.

Naproxen is effective in all of the inflammatory arthritides and in both osteoarthritis and non-articular rheumatism and it is usually well tolerated. It exerts an analgesic effect at least equal to that of the standard analgesic drugs such as paracetamol or dextropropoxyphene. Again, individual patients fail to respond, but it is not possible to predict this in advance.

Adverse reactions may involve the upper gastrointestinal tract (by far the most common) or the central nervous system. Headaches, confusion or depression may occur, but these may appear with all the first line drugs. Early fears of massive gastrointestinal haemorrhage have been put into perspective, being exceedingly rare. In common with most of these drugs, naproxen may produce sodium retention with all its implications, especially in the elderly and in those with compromised renal function; in addition, it will produce interference in tests for the estimation of urinary 17-ketogenic steroids and 5-hydroxyindoleacetic acid.

Naproxen is prescribed as yellow tablets (250 or 500 mg), and a 500 mg suppository is available. The dose varies between 500 mg and 1.5 g in accordance with patient preference and some patients prefer the b.d. option made available by its long half-life. Naproxen sodium is a separately marketed alternative with little to commend it in a strictly medical context.

Flurbiprofen

Flurbiprofen [2-(2-fluoro-4-biphenyl)propionic acid], is a compound which shares most of the properties described above in the context of the other propionic acid drugs. It is rapidly absorbed after oral administration, peak plasma concentrations being achieved within 1–2 h of ingestion. The plasma half-life is of the order of 3–4 h and there is no accumulation. The drug penetrates slowly into the synovium. Steady-state concentrations are achieved within 7 days of regular administration. The drug is transported bound to albumin to the liver, where it is metabolised, subsequently to be excreted through the renal tubular cell. Antirheumatic activity of this drug resides in the parent molecule and not in its metabolites. Although it is firmly bound to albumin, it occupies only 10% of the binding sites—hence it has less potential to displace other drugs. Before instituting such a regimen, however, it is wise to question the need for each drug in accordance with normal practice.

Flurbiprofen is an effective antirheumatic drug and has been used widely in all varieties of inflammatory and non-inflammatory diseases. It is no more toxic than the other members of this group and again it is patient preference which dictates its selection. The main adverse reactions encountered have been gastrointestinal in nature but they are not predictable. Flurbiprofen has been administered without harm in patients who had proven peptic ulceration, as indeed have all of the other members of this group of drugs, but caution is required.

Flurbiprofen is available as 50 and 100 mg tablets and the dose varies between 200 mg and 300 mg.

Fenbufen

Fenbufen is a biphenylpropionic acid which has two metabolites which are themselves highly active and thus prolong the effect of this drug, allowing it to be prescribed on a once-a-day basis. One of these (4-biphenylacetic acid) is chemically similar to diclofenac.

Fenbufen, which has properties very similar to those of the other propionic acids, has been studied extensively in field trials. The dose recommended at present is 600 or 900 mg taken late at night, but in the light of experience with all of the other drugs of this class it is likely that this will be modified in the future. Two new propionic drugs, tiaprofenic acid and indoprofen, have properties similar to the drugs mentioned above.

Phenylacetic Acids

Fenclofenac

Fenclofenac [2-(2,4-dichlorophenoxy)phenylacetic acid] is a weakly acidic arylacetic acid which is well absorbed after oral administration. The biological half-life is 18–24 h permitting a b.d. dosage. The arylacetic acids share many properties with the propionic acids in vitro and in animal models and are effective analgesic, antipyretic and anti-inflammatory compounds. They inhibit prostaglandin synthetases and have a similar array of other biological effects.

Fenclofenac peak plasma concentrations occur within 1 h of ingestion of an oral dose, and equilibrium is reached within 7–10 days of regular administration. This compound is transported bound to plasma proteins and is metabolised in the hepatocyte, subsequently to be excreted through the renal tubules. It is claimed that the differences between the intermediary metabolism of this and of the closely related compound, diclofenac, are responsible for the differences in the spectrum of side-effects. Fenclofenac is more likely to produce a skin rash whereas diclofenac produces its main toxicity in the gastrointestinal tract. The skin rash begins as a maculopapular eruption which may be distributed widely over the trunk and limbs. It usually begins within 10–14 days of starting treatment and may become very severe with evidence of underlying vasculitis and constitutional involvement. If the drug is stopped promptly the eruption usually fades slowly, in severe cases with desquamation. The only other adverse reaction which is encountered commonly is dyspepsia. Fenclofenac will produce a profound disturbance in thyroid function tests.

The dose lies between 0.6 and 1.2 g per day in divided doses in proportion to the patient's age, weight and disease.

Suggestions that fenclofenac may produce an additional disease-modifying effect in rheumatoid arthritis have been advanced by the company concerned but should be viewed with caution and suspicion at the moment.

Diclofenac

Diclofenac [(2,6-dichlorophenyl)-aminophenylacetic acid] is presented as the sodium salt and shares common properties with the other arylacetic acids. It is absorbed well from the gastrointestinal tract after oral administration and is transported, bound to plasma albumin, to the liver. There is an enterohepatic recirculation and after metabolism to water-soluble derivatives in the hepatocyte, excretion occurs through the renal tubule. Ninety-five per cent of the administered dose may be recovered in the urine within 96 h of ingestion.

Peak plasma concentrations occur within 30 min to 1 h after ingestion, slightly later in the case of the enteric-coated preparation. Because of the enterohepatic recirculation there is a biphasic metabolism, the second peak appearing 1.5–2.5 h after ingestion. It takes up to 2 weeks of regular administration before equilibrium is achieved.

Diclofenac penetrates the synovial membrane slowly and thereafter concentrations in synovial fluid exceed those of paired plasma samples. Complex interactions with other drugs may occur. In the case of aspirin, diclofenac will displace aspirin from its albumin binding site but aspirin in turn will interfere with enterohepatic recirculation, tending to reduce the plasma concentration of diclofenac. The binding constant of diclofenac to albumin is high and diclofenac will displace warfarin, sulphonylureas and hydantoins. In renal failure the biliary excretion route may be expanded, tending to oppose a rise in plasma concentration. As with any newly introduced drug, however, caution is mandatory for the first few years of use at least.

There seems to be little doubt that diclofenac is an effective antirheumatic drug and field studies have been conducted in all of the inflammatory arthritides and in osteoarthritis, degenerative disc disease and non-articular rheumatism. The drug seems to have been well tolerated, the most frequent adverse reactions encountered to date being gastrointestinal in nature. Central nervous system side-effects with headaches and confusion have been reported and there have been some skin rashes. One patient who developed the Stevens-Johnson syndrome has been reported. Anaemia and abnormal liver function tests have also been documented. "Aspirin asthma" may occur.

A dose regimen of 50 mg three times per day reducing to 25 mg three times per day has been recommended.

Indenes

Sulindac

Sulindac [(Z)-5-fluoro-2-methyl-1-(p-(methylsulphinyl)phenyl methylene-1H-indene-3-acetic acid], is a methylated indenedione, the indene differing from the indole configuration of indomethacin. It is a stable yellow compound soluble in water at neutral and alkaline pH. Removal of the fluorine from C5 destroys its analgesic properties. The centre of metabolism is the methylsulphinyl structure, which may be oxidised, yielding a sulphone and a sulphide. The sulphide, which has a long biological half-life and is strongly bound to albumin, is the biologically active moeity. It is this compound which inhibits prostaglandin synthetase.

Sulindac is promptly absorbed from the gastrointestinal tract and is transported bound to plasma protein, being metabolised in the hepatocyte. There is a marked enterohepatic recirculation and sulindac is metabolised further in the gastrointestinal tract to the sulphide, which is then reabsorbed. The sulphone and glucuronide metabolites are excreted through the renal tubule.

Following absorption, peak plasma concentrations appear within 1 h in the case of the parent molecule and at 2 h for the active sulphide. The half-life of sulindac is between 7 and 8 h and the half-life of the sulphide derivative is between 16 and 18 h. There is a constant ratio of sulindac to the sulphide.

Sulindac is effective in the treatment of a wide variety of different arthritides. The principal adverse reactions encountered to date are gastrointestinal and central nervous system side-effects and skin rashes. Headaches, confusion and depression may all occur, and "allergic" asthmatic reactions are possible with this as with aspirin and many of the other first line drugs. The recommended dose is 200 mg b.d.

It is becoming increasingly apparent that drugs with prolonged half-lives must be viewed with particular circumspection; therefore additional caution should be exercised before and during the prescription of proposed new NSAIDs such as sulindac.

Oxicams

Piroxicam

The oxicams are a different class of drugs. Piroxicam is a product of four separate chemical groups, each of which conveys a different property upon the final product. It is a 4-hydroxy-1,2-benzothiouric,4-hydroxy-2-methyl-N-(2-pyridyl)-2H,1,2-benzothiozine 11-dioxide. It is an acid by virtue of the enolization of the 4-hydroxy substitution.

Piroxicam has analgesic, antipyretic and anti-inflammatory properties in animal models. Its mode of action is not corticosteroid dependent but it does inhibit prostaglandin synthetases. It also inhibits the motility of mononuclear phagocytes and the aggregation of platelets.

Piroxicam is rapidly and smoothly absorbed from the small intestine. It has a half-life of 38 h, permitting once a day dosage. The drug is transported to the liver, where hydroxylation of the pyridyl ring is followed by conjugation with glucuronic acid. The water-soluble metabolites are excreted through the renal tubular cells.

As with sulindac, it must be constantly remembered that this drug has a long half-life.

Pyrazolones

Phenylbutazone

Phenylbutazone [1,2-diphenyl 3,5 dioxo-4-N-butylpyrazolidine] is a lipophylic, moderately acidic compound which was introduced in 1949. There is no doubt that it is a highly effective antirheumatic drug and the criticisms should be directed at its clinical abuse rather that at the molecule.

It is an effective and powerful antipyretic, analgesic and anti-inflammatory drug which also produces sodium retention and uricosuria. It is a prostaglandin synthetase inhibitor and stabilises biological membranes. It uncouples oxidative phosphorylation and interferes with a wide variety of different enzymes.

Absorption from the small intestine is rapid, and peak plasma concentrations appear within 2–3 h of ingestion. It circulates bound to plasma proteins and will displace other protein-bound drugs. Phenylbutazone has a long half-life (48–54 h) and penetrates the blood-brain and the placental barrier and the synovial membrane. One of its principal metabolites, oxyphenylbutazone, also possesses anti-inflammatory properties. Absorption of phenylbutazone is inhibited by concurrent prescription of tricyclic antidepressants. The drug is transported to the liver and excreted following metabolic transformation through the renal tubule.

The side-effects of phenylbutazone (and of oxyphenylbutazone) are the limiting factor to its prescription. Gastrointestinal intolerance is the most common and may be reduced but not abolished by enteric coating and by taking the tablet with meals. Acute erosions may be produced and phenylbutazone may exacerbate an established peptic ulcer. Skin rashes of all varieties and all severities may occur, including the Stevens-Johnson syndrome, and may be related to the pyrazolidine ring since they also occur with other drugs which possess this configuration. Jaundice of both the obstructive and the hepatitic type may be produced and goitre may develop as a result of interference with the intrathyroidal organification process. Microscopic haematuria may be produced and there is a rare syndrome associated with phenylbutazone where the patient presents with lymphadenopathy, hepatosplenomegaly and salivary gland enlargement. A much more common drawback of phenylbutazone therapy, particularly in the elderly and in those with impairment of cardiac reserve, is the precipitation of congestive cardiac failure on the basis of sodium retention.

By far the most alarming adverse reaction with phenylbutazone is its effects upon the haematological system. Agranulocytosis occurs in the young after brief exposure whereas aplastic anaemia is more likely to present in the elderly following prolonged treatment. This is an additional reason why phenylbutazone should most certainly never be prescribed for the elderly. Thrombocytopenia may present acutely alone or may form part of aplastic anaemia. The haematological adverse reactions may develop slowly or appear precipitously. Thus although regular blood counts are important, if only for medicolegal reasons, they should not induce complacency. The most culpable situation is where a young person, prescribed phenylbutazone or oxyphenylbutazone for a minor sports injury, develops agranulocytosis and dies. This, in a situation where there are so many perfectly adequate alternatives, is totally unacceptable medical practice. Even worse is the practice of prescribing combination medication incorporating both phenylbutazone and corticosteroid. Forty persons in the United Kingdom died last year as a result of the clinical abuse of this drug.

Phenylbutazone should be viewed as a second line drug and should only be prescribed in the circumstance of failure of general measures and a single first line drug. When prescribed in this way with full appreciation of the risks then phenylbutazone remains a very valuable drug and may have a special role as a second line drug in patients with the seronegative spondarthritides.

In the light of its long half-life a once-a-day regimen is feasible. Both some side-effects and efficacy display a dose-response relationship, 300 mg per day producing greater clinical benefit than 50 mg per day. As always, the dose should be kept to a minimum.

Benzotriazines

Azapropazone

Azapropazone   [3-demethylamino-7-methyl-1,2(n-propylmalonyl)1,2-dihydro-2,4-benzotriazine dihydrate] is a condensation product of benzotriazine with a pyrazolidine ring. It is a yellow odourless compound which is slightly soluble in acid and more so in alkaline medium.

It has analgesic, antipyretic and anti-inflammatory properties in animal models of inflammatory arthritis and will inhibit prostaglandins as well as a wide array of other enzymes. It will also stabilise lysosomal and other cell membranes. It has antibradykinin activity and is uricosuric. It will inhibit the motility of mononuclear phagocytic cells and reduce vascular permeability.

Azapropazone is well absorbed from the small intestine and there is a pronounced enterohepatic recirculation resulting in complex peak plasma concentration graphs. The plasma half-life is 12 h but the biological half-life is prolonged to values in the range of 20 h. Equilibrium is attained after 7–10 days of regular administration. The drug is tightly bound to plasma proteins and will displace other protein-bound drugs; it is hydroxylated in the hepatocyte to an inactive metabolite. A large proportion is excreted through the renal tubules as the parent molecule (more than 70%) and the rest as the hydroxylated metabolite. The implication of this is that caution must be exercised in patients with impaired renal function since so much of the active material depends upon intact renal function for its excretion.

This drug is an effective antirheumatic compound and has been tested in a wide array of different clinical situations. The dose recommended at present is 1200–1800 mg per day on a b.d. basis, and it is suggested that caution be exercised in patients with active peptic ulceration or with renal impairment. It will interfere with anticoagulants, anticonvulsants and oral antidiabetic agents.

The adverse reactions encountered to date include gastrointestinal upset, skin rashes, headache, confusion, depression and fluid retention. One major anxiety, engendered by its molecular similarity to phenylbutazone, namely the possibility of haematological side-effects, has not yet proved to be well founded.

Further Reading

Akyol S, Thompson M, Kerr DNS (1982) Renal function after prolonged aspirin consumption. Br Med J 284: 631–632

Bernstein BN, Singsen BH, King KK, Hanson V (1977) Aspirin induced hepatotoxicity and its effect on juvenile rheumatoid arthritis. Am J Dis Child 131: 659–663

Brooks PM, Bell MA, Sturrock RD, Famaey JP, Dick WC (1974) The clinical significance of indomethacin-probenecid interaction. Br J Clin Pharmacol 1: 287–290

Brooks PM, Bell MA, Lee P, Rooney PJ, Dick WC (1974) The effect of frusemide on indomethacin plasma levels. Br J Clin Pharmacol 1: 485–489

Capell HA, Rennie JAN, Rooney PJ, Murdoch RM, Hole DJ, Dick WC, Buchanan WW (1979) Patient compliance; a novel method of testing nonsteroidal antiinflammatory analgesics in rheumatoid arthritis. J Rheumatol 6: 584–593

Dick WC (1977) Drug treatment of rheumatoid arthritis. In: Scott JT (ed) Copeman's textbook of the rheumatic diseases, 5th edn. Churchill Livingstone, Edinburgh London New York, Chap 16

Dunk AA, Walt RP, Jenkins WJ, Sherlock SS (1982) Diclofenac hepatitis. Br Med J 284: 1605–1606

Eknoyn G, Qunibi WY, Grisson RT, Tuma SN, Ayms JC (1982) Renal papillary necrosis—an update. Medicine 61: 55–73

Fowler PD, Faragher EB (1977) Drug and nondrug factors influencing adverse reactions to pyrazoles. J Int Med Res 5(2): 108–120

Goldstein J, Laskin D, Ginsberg G (1980) Sulindac associated pancreatitis. Ann Intern Med 83: 151

Goodman WS, Gillman AC (1980) The pharmacological basis of therapeutics, 6th edn. Macmillan, New York

Goodwin JS, Regan M (1982) Cognitive dysfunction associated with naproxen and ibuprofen in the elderly. Arthritis Rheum 25: 1013–1015

Hart FD (1979) Drug treatment of the rheumatic diseases. Adis Health Science Press, Sydney

Kowanko IC, Pownall R, Knapp MS, Swannell AJ, Mahoney PGC (1981) Circadian variations in the signs and symptoms of rheumatoid arthritis and in the therapeutic effectiveness of Flurbiprofen at different times of the day. Br J Clin Pharmacol 11: 477–484

Northover BJ (1977) Indomethacin—a calcium antagonist. Gen Pharmacol 8: 293–296

Quigley MR, Richfield M, Krumlovsky FA, Kanwar YS, Carone FA, Jarrett MP (1982) Concurrent naproxen and penicillamine induced renal disease in rheumatoid arthritis. Arthritis Rheum 25: 1016–1019

Rumble RH, Brooks PM, Roberts MS (1980) Metabolism of salicylate during chronic aspirin therapy. Br J Pharmacol 9: 41–45

Segre EJ, Chaplin M, Forchiella E, Runkel R, Sevelius H (1973) Naproxen–aspirin interactions in man. Clin Pharmacol Ther 374–379

Taylor R, Clarke F, Griffiths IDG, Weeke J (1980) Prospective study of the effect of Fenclofenac on thyroid function tests. Br Med J 281: 911–912

15 Gold

History

It is somewhat sobering to write about gold therapy in the 1980s when as long ago as 1927 Lande drew attention to its possible role in the treatment of rheumatoid arthritis. Robert Koch reported the inhibition of growth of tubercle bacilli by gold compounds in 1890, and early twentieth century physicians used gold in rheumatoid arthritis, believing the pathology to be similar to that of tuberculosis. Lande's observation was substantiated by Forester in 1929, but it was not until 1945 that a controlled double-blind study was reported by Fraser from Glasgow. Despite essentially favourable results from this study, acceptance of gold therapy in rheumatoid arthritis only became widespread after the report of the Empire Rheumatism Council in 1960, which again demonstrated its superiority over placebo. It is interesting to speculate that the proper study of gold as a therapeutic regimen might have been retarded by the dramatic introduction of corticosteroids in 1948, which overshadowed the use of other drugs for many years.

Subsequent publications have validated these early studies on the value of gold in the treatment of patients with rheumatoid arthritis and recently it has been suggested that in responding patients gold fundamentally alters the natural history of the disease. However, many questions about the mode of action and best method of prescription of gold compounds remain unanswered and provide a fertile field for rheumatological research.

More recently oral gold compounds have been studied. These are at present still under investigation and this chapter will deal primarily with intramuscular gold therapy.

Chemistry

Gold exists in monovalent and trivalent forms, both of which will avidly complex with ligands. Therapeutic compounds are aurous salts in which gold is attached to sulphydryl sulphur. Gold has a strong affinity for sulphur and an inhibitory effect on pyruvic dehydrogenase. These properties have led to the suggestion that the therapeutic effect of gold salts may be due in part to inhibition of sulphydryl systems, although not all sulphydryl inhibitors exhibit a similar effect.

Gold has a low chemical reactivity and gold compounds tend to decompose to the elemental form. Thiol compounds are used since they are more stable and the water-soluble preparations contain hydrophilic groups in addition to the aurothio group.

It is possible that the thiol groups exert activity in their own right and this is being investigated at the moment in Oslo.

Pharmacological Actions

This brief outline of pharmacological actions refers to sodium auriothiomalate, although some of the actions described are common to other gold compounds.

Animal work has unfortunately contributed little in this sphere except in the dissection of the pathogenesis of renal side-effects and will not be discussed here. In the rheumatoid patient sodium aurothiomalate probably acts at many sites in the inflammatory response which leads to tissue damage. Prostaglandin synthesis is inhibited, vascular permeability is decreased and there are fewer cells at inflammatory sites. Cell migration and chemotaxis are suppressed along with phagocytic action and lysosomal enzyme activity. There is an interaction with sulphydryl groups and inactivation of sulphydryl-dependent enzymes may be relevant therapeutically.

The effect of gold on the immune response is complex and in vivo the most consistent changes are related to B-lymphocytic function. Rheumatoid factor titres fall and over a period of several years immunoglobulins diminish. The effect on T-lymphocytic function is less clear, and while altered cell-mediated immunity and inhibition of complement activation can be demonstrated in vitro, it is not known if these are relevant in vivo. Albumin levels increase during gold therapy and there is an effect on trace metals, particularly copper and zinc. The latter effect and the role of superoxide dismutase require further clarification.

Absorption, Distribution and Excretion

After intramuscular injection of sodium aurothiomalate a peak serum gold level is obtained within 2 h, and the concentration declines gradually over the ensuing week. During the first 6–8 weeks of weekly injections of 50 mg there is a slow increase in the gold concentration which then reaches a plateau, providing dose and frequency of injection remain constant.

Gold diffuses rapidly between serum and synovial fluid and reaches equilibrium within hours of an intramuscular injection. It is possible to measure gold concentrations in protein fractions by carbon furnace atomic absorption spectrometry, and most of the 92% of gold which is protein bound is in the albumin fraction. Plasma and serum gold levels do not correlate with efficacy or toxicity. Gold can also be identified in urine, but again these levels do not correlate with clinical benefit or adverse reactions.

Gold particles can be demonstrated in the cornea in a concentration proportional to the cumulative gold dose. This deposition reverses when gold therapy is stopped and does not produce ocular toxicity.

Of the gold which accumulates in skin, 3% is in the epidermis and 97% in the dermis. Gold particles have been identified in lysosomes of dermal histiocytes.

Between 30% and 53% of administered gold is excreted each week, mostly in the urine. The rate of excretion is not helpful in predicting toxicity.

Indications

Rheumatoid Arthritis

Gold remains one of the most useful drugs for the management of active rheumatoid arthritis which is leading to progressive destruction of joints. Selection of patients is discussed in detail in Chap. 13.

The only gold preparation currently available in the United Kingdom is sodium aurothiomalate (Myocrisin, May and Baker).

Studies comparing aqueous aurothiomalate and oil-based aurothioglucose (Solganal), both of which are available in the United States, have generally failed to show a significant difference between the two preparations. Oral gold compounds are currently being studied.

The therapeutic regimen for gold therapy varies greatly in different centres but a suggested treatment schedule is to administer 50 mg weekly following a 10 mg test dose. If the patient responds, the interval between injections is increased to 2 and then 3 weeks and ultimately a maintenance dose of 50 mg is given every 4–6 weeks; if no response is witnessed after administration of 1000 mg, one might try (a) 100 mg weekly for 5 weeks or (b) another second line drug.

There is no evidence that tailoring the dose to individual weight or to plasma levels confers any advantage. It has been suggested that a weekly dose of 25 mg or even 10 mg is as effective as 50 mg, but since these studies have failed to show diminished toxicity many rheumatologists continue to use a 50 mg weekly dose.

If no serious side-effects are encountered and benefit has been obtained, maintenance gold is continued indefinitely at 4–6 weekly intervals. This is recommended even when remission has been substantial and where non-steroidal anti-inflammatory drugs have become superfluous. The experience of earlier studies where only a "course" of gold was used and of patients who default from follow up because they feel so well, is of relapse after a variable period. Similarly, patients who have responded but who have had therapy withdrawn because of side-effects almost invariably relapse.

Perhaps less understandable is the late relapse which may occur after an initially good remission and despite adherence to maintenance therapy. Attempts to recapture the effect by increasing the frequency and/or the dose of injections are usually unsuccessful. Nevertheless, it is probably justifiable to try this approach before abandoning gold therapy, since occasional patients do respond.

Blood, urine, skin and mucous membranes should be checked at the time of each injection. If the white cell count is less than 4000 per cm^3 or platelet count less than 150 000 per cm^3 (both these are the lower limit of normal in our laboratory), gold should be withheld while the count is checked. A sudden confirmed fall dictates permanent cessation of therapy.

If there is more than a trace of protein on dipstix, gold is withheld while urine is cultured and a 24-h urinary protein level estimated. Confirmation of significant proteinuria (>300 mg/24 h) without an alternative explanation means that gold needs to be discontinued until proteinuria clears, after which cautious reintroduction may be attempted. Prolonged significant proteinuria should be investigated by renal biopsy and gold should not be reintroduced after the occurrence of nephrotic range proteinuria. Gold therapy should cease temporarily if rash or mouth ulceration occur, even if a definite causal relationship is impossible to establish. When these mucocutaneous side- effects have settled, a further attempt at treatment may be made. Where severe rash has occurred, however, such an attempt is inadvisable.

Psoriatic Arthropathy

In the past gold therapy has been considered more toxic and less effective in patients with psoriatic arthropathy. However, a recent report (Dorwart et al. 1978) showed efficacy in psoriatic arthritis. This awaits confirmation in other studies from other centres.

Complications

Gold toxicity has engendered considerable anxiety over the 50 years it has been used in the treatment of rheumatoid arthritis. While it is true that inappropriate dosage and monitoring has in the past created a somewhat false impression, gold remains a potentially toxic drug. If sustained supervision is not possible, gold should not be used.

Bone Marrow

Gold has been reported as a cause of agranulocytosis, thrombocytopaenia, total marrow aplasia and, more rarely, pure red cell aplasia. Haematological complications are uncommon but the exact incidence is difficult to ascertain, especially against a background of rheumatological polypharmacy.

Granulocytopaenia/Agranulocytosis. This complication may be detected on routine testing or occasionally may present with pharyngitis and fever. Granulocytopaenia usually reverses on withdrawal of gold but a further trial of gold therapy is not justified. If there are fewer than 1000 neutrophils our policy is to admit the patient to a laminar flow haematology unit where full bacteriological screening is maintained until the count has risen. Any infection is treated promptly and prophylactic nasal and bowel sterilisation is routine.

Thrombocytopaenia. Occasionally a gradual fall in platelets is observed and this reverses on cessation of gold therapy. More alarming (and slightly more frequent) is a precipitous fall in platelets from a normal count one week to less than 20000 the next. Even meticulous monitoring will not anticipate this complication, and the patient may present with purpura only a few days after a normal platelet count. Management in this instance is supportive. A brief period of high dose (40–60 mg) prednisolone is given and if the risk of bleeding is high, platelet transfusions should be administered even though transfused platelet survival time will be short. Platelets usually return to normal over 7–10 days and prednisolone can then be reduced and finally stopped. Very occasionally platelets fail to return to normal levels and splenectomy has been used in some reported cases.

Renal

Proteinuria with or without haematuria may occur during gold therapy. The relationship of these abnormalities to treatment has been debated and certainly the renal complications of rheumatoid arthritis itself and of non- steroidal anti-inflammatory drug therapy are ill understood. Nevertheless, gold is implicated in the development of a membranous glomerulonephritis which reverses on withdrawal of therapy. Tubular necrosis may also occur.

The reported frequency of renal abnormalities during gold therapy varies greatly. Transient proteinuria is fairly common while severe proteinuria in the nephrotic range is rare. There is no relationship to blood or urine levels of gold, and the unpredictable dose range required to produce proteinuria suggests hypersensitivity. A few cases described in the literature have subsequently been shown to have SLE.

Pathologically and histologically (light and electron microscopically) gold inclusions can be demonstrated in glomerular and tubular epithelial cells in patients who are on gold therapy. In those patients who develop gold toxicity, electron-dense subepithelial basement membrane deposits are found, the nature of which is uncertain. These are reminiscent of idiopathic glomerular nephritis, and on immunofluorescence stain intensively with antisera against IgG, IgM and C3. The presence of immunoglobulins and complement along the basement membrane may occur as a result of glomerular damage and does not necessarily imply existence of an immune complex mechanism. It is becoming more and more likely that the mechanisms of production of both gold and penicillamine nephropathy are similar. Interesting and important results are being obtained at present in the study of gold and heavy metal nephropathy in the Brown Norwegian rat.

Proteinuria usually reverses over a period of months following gold withdrawal and only supportive treatment and exclusion of other causes is required. Even patients with the nephrotic syndrome appear to have a good prognosis, but if proteinuria persists, amyloidosis should be suspected and renal biopsy undertaken.

Postinjection Reactions

Vasomotor (Nitritoid). Symptoms of facial flushing, weakness, sweating and occasional fainting do occur following gold sodium thiomalate injections and are usually mild and transient. There may be associated nausea and vomiting and a sinus tachycardia may be observed. These reactions are said not to occur with gold thioglucose but when this alternative is not available, reassurance and perseverance will usually allow gold therapy to be continued. These reactions emphasise the importance of adhering strictly to the practice of prescribing a 10 mg test injection before commencing a gold regimen.

Non-vasomotor. Transient stiffness, arthralgia and myalgia with or without constitutional symptoms and occurring within 24 h of gold sodium thiomalate injections are reported by some patients. This reaction may be under- reported by patients accustomed to variation in disease severity or expecting to experience a different effect from a drug described as potentially toxic. A mechanism whereby gold temporarily inhibits reticuloendothelial function in these patients has been postulated but not proven. It is important that gold therapy should not be abandoned prematurely in these patients since they are as likely to respond to therapy as patients without postinjection reactions. Again, substitution of gold thioglucose is said to prevent the reaction but this option is not universally available.

Skin and Mucous Membranes

Skin. Rashes associated with gold therapy may occur at any time and at any site. Pruritus, which may antedate the appearance of the rash, is characteristic. An early generalised maculopapular rash may develop but does not necessarily recur if gold is tried again. Later rashes present with lesions which are often discrete, scaly and erythematous and will settle if gold is withheld. Exfoliative dermatitis which was described in the older literature should not now occur providing the importance of a cautious approach is recognised. Symptomatic treatment for pruritus is sometimes helpful.

Mucous Membranes. Oral ulceration, and more rarely ulceration of genital mucous membrane, can be a troublesome side-effect of gold. Chrysotherapy should not be given in the presence of stomatitis but may be restarted at a lower dose once ulceration has healed.

Chrysiasis. Deposition of gold in skin may lead to diffuse darkening in light-exposed areas. This side-effect is apparently dose related. Similarly, gold deposition in the cornea may produce corneal chrysiasis, which is asymptomatic and disappears after withdrawal of gold.

Hepatotoxicity

Relatively few cases of hepatitis have been described recently and it is possible that many early reports could now be ascribed to other causes, in particular the reuse of infected needles. Nevertheless, cholestatic hepatitis is a potential, albeit unusual, complication in patients treated with gold, and may appear at low doses (in one case report intrahepatic cholestasis developed in an 8-year-old boy after only two injections totalling 35 mg gold sodium thiomalate). The abnormalities of hepatic function reverse completely when gold is withheld, and rechallenge is not justifiable.

Gastrointestinal

Enterocolitis in association with gold therapy is exceedingly rare, and since not all reported cases had definite or classical rheumatoid arthritis, the underlying diagnosis of inflammatory bowel disease with associated arthropathy could not be excluded.

Three of six reported cases occurred in Israel and a genetic predisposition (or local awareness) may be relevant. The dose of gold administered prior to onset of diarrhoea was small, and the outcome fatal in most cases. It would thus seem prudent to regard the occurrence of diarrhoea in patients on gold seriously and to withhold therapy until another reason for the diarrhoea has been found and treated. It is possible that this may prove to be a greater problem with oral gold regimens.

Pulmonary Involvement

The occurrence of pulmonary fibrosis and infiltrates in association with gold therapy has been reported but a causal relationship is not proven. In the published cases withdrawal of gold has coincided with clearing of pulmonary lesions.

Neuropathy

Cases of peripheral neuropathy considered attributable to chrysotherapy have been reported.

Genetic Predisposition to Gold Toxicity

It has been suggested that patients with DR3 are particularly likely to develop proteinuria and haematological side-effects on gold. The association of a particular haplotype with gold and with penicillamine toxicity is an important and fascinating observation which raises many questions in terms of both research and clinical practice. These questions are being investigated intensively at present.

Use of Gold in Pregnancy

Gold is contraindicated in pregnancy but may need to be resumed postpartum.

Summary

Gold remains a valuable drug in the management of moderate to severe rheumatoid arthritis. Well supervised, the co-operative patient may derive considerable benefit. Poor monitoring increases toxicity to an unacceptable level.

Further Reading

Co-operating Clinics Committee of the American Rheumatism Association (1973) A controlled trial of gold salt therapy in rheumatoid arthritis. Arthritis Rheum 16: 353–358

Dorwart BB, Gall EP, Schumacher HR, Klauser RE (1978) Chrysotherapy in psoriatic arthritis. Arthritis Rheum 21: 513–515

Hinglais H, Druet P, Grossetete J, Sapin C, Bariety J (1979) Ultrastructural study of nephritis induced in brown Norway rats by mercuric chloride. Lab Invest 41(2): 150–159

Hunneyball IM (1980) Recent developments in disease modifying antirheumatic drugs. Prog Drug Res 24: 101–216

Kean WF, Lock CJL, Howard-Lock HE, Buchanan WW (1982) Prior gold therapy does not influence the adverse effects of D-penicillamine in rheumatoid arthritis. Arthritis Rheum 25: 917–922

Research Sub-committee of the Empire Rheumatism Council (1960) Gold therapy in rheumatoid arthritis. Ann Rheum Dis 19: 95–119

Scott DL, Bradby GVH, Aitman TJ, Zaphiropolos GC, Hawkins CF (1981) Relationship of gold and penicillamine therapy to diffuse interstitial lung disease. Ann Rheum Dis 40: 580–583

Sigler JW, Bluhm GB et al. (1974) Gold salts in the treatment of rheumatoid arthritis. Ann Rheum Dis 80: 21–26

Silverberg DS, Kidd EG, Shnitkn TK, Ulan RA (1970) Gold nephropathy: A clinical and pathological study. Arthritis Rheum 13: 812–825

Srinivasan R, Millar B, Paulus H (1979) Long term chrysotherapy in rheumatoid arthritis. Arthr Rheum 22: 105–110

Tornroth T, Skrifuars B (1974) Gold nephropathy prototype of membranous glomerulonephritis. Am J Pathol 75: 573–588

Vaamonde CA, Hunt FR (1970) The nephrotic syndrome as a complication of gold therapy. Arthritis Rheum 13: 826–834

Wooley JC, Griffen J, Panayi GS, Batchelor JR, Welsh KI, Gibson TJ (1980) HLA Dr antigens and toxic reactions to sodium aurothiomalate and D-penicillamine in patients with rheumatoid arthritis. N Engl J Med 303: 300–302

16 Penicillamine

History

Penicillamine was first used therapeutically by Walshe, who recognised and utilised its cupruretic effect in 1956, thus revolutionising the management of hepatolenticular degeneration. The actual isolation of penicillamine, a crystalline degradation product of penicillin, had occurred some 13 years earlier, when Abraham and his co-workers were studying the chemistry of penicillin.

The use of penicillamine in rheumatoid arthritis was based on a hypothesis which was subsequently not substantiated. Jaffe postulated that the in vitro capacity of penicillamine to cleave macroglobulin linkages might be used against rheumatoid factor and thus arrest the disease process. Short courses of systemic therapy did not produce clinical improvement, nor did intra-articular injection of penicillamine. However, Jaffe was able to show significant improvement in symptoms of patients with rheumatoid arthritis when the treatment period was extended to several months. Although rheumatoid factor titres were reduced by penicillamine, clinical improvement antedated this reduction. The mode of action was unclear but an important clinical effect had been demonstrated in rheumatoid disease, and this was later confirmed by other observers and by a multicentre double–blind study. Toxicity was greater than in Wilson's disease or cystinuria (where benefit had also been conclusively demonstrated) but overall efficacy was found to be similar to gold.

More recently the use of "go low—go slow" regimens has partially reduced toxicity. However, during extended use of the drug a number of adverse reactions have been attributed to penicillamine therapy.

Chemistry

Penicillamine is a trifunctional amino acid which differs from cysteine in that the hydrogen atoms at the C-3 atom are replaced by two methyl groups. It is thus designated 3,3-dimethylcysteine, and may exist as the D or L stereoisomer. The L isomer is extremely toxic and penicillamine as used today (which may be derived from the controlled hydrolysis of penicillin or wholly synthesised) consists only of the D isomer.

Biochemical Actions

1. *Sulphydryl–disulphide exchange*: Penicillamine is a reducing agent for the disulphide bonds of many proteins.
2. *Metal chelation*: Penicillamine will form complexes of varying stability with metals such as nickel, copper, mercury, lead, zinc, cobalt, iron and manganese. The D-penicillamine–copper complex has been shown to possess superoxide dismutase activity.
3. *Thiazolidine formation*: A thiazolidine derivative capable of displacing amino acids is formed when penicillamine reacts with pyridoxal-5-phosphate.

The relevance of the above three types of reactions to the therapeutic activity of penicillamine in rheumatoid arthritis is unclear.
   Penicillamine is more stable than cysteine, being less readily oxidised. Unlike cysteine, therefore, it is not rapidly converted to the disulphide in vivo and this is of value therapeutically.

Absorption, Distribution and Excretion

Pharmacodynamic studies of penicillamine have until recently been limited because of the difficulty in attaching a radioactive label to a product of fermentation. There has thus been no satisfactory way of measuring the drug in blood and tissues. However, studies done with ^{35}S-labelled synthetic DL-penicillamine in patients with Wilson's disease have shown peak plasma concentrations within 1–2 h of ingestion. Clearance fell rapidly after 4 h and by 48 h 1% of the label was still present on plasma and was mainly protein bound. Most of the ^{35}S label appeared in blood or urine as free penicillamine or penicillamine–cysteine mixed disulphide with small amounts of intermediates.
   The following points have been elucidated in connection with the metabolism of penicillamine:

1. Penicillamine is rapidly absorbed from the gastrointestinal tract, although a proportion is unabsorbed and may be degraded in the gut.
2. It is widely distributed throughout the body water space and excreted by the kidney until plasma protein and tissue binding reduce the rate of clearance.

3. It is metabolically inert.

4. Part of a dose persists in the body in a reduced form or as a disulphide for long periods (the bound fraction will survive as long as its carrier protein) despite the rapid initial urinary excretion.

5. Using liquid chromatography and an electrochemical detector it is now possible to measure total plasma penicillamine (reduced+disulphide).

In the past most studies were conducted in rats, human volunteers, cystinurics (where, for example, urinary excretion differs) or patients with Wilson's disease. The techniques mentioned under point 5 above have recently been used in rheumatoid patients and should facilitate detailed studies of penicillamine pharmacokinetics in these patients. Such studies may enable clinicians to use the drug with greater efficacy and diminished toxicity (although gold kinetic studies have proved disappointing in this connection).

Rheumatological Indications and Use

Rheumatoid Arthritis

Progressive erosive rheumatoid arthritis, is the most common rheumatological indication for the use of penicillamine. In controlled studies penicillamine has been shown to produce significant improvement in articular index, duration of morning stiffness, pain score, walking time, grip strength, ESR and rheumatoid factor when compared with placebo. Response occurs over several months and resembles that achieved with chrysotherapy. General approach and contraindications to its use are as outlined in Chap. 13. One of the major problems of penicillamine compared with intramuscular gold is that patients will obtain a supply of the drug and thus may be able to manipulate their own dose with potentially disastrous results. Education about the importance of regular monitoring and adherence to the prescribed regimen is mandatory. If the willingness or ability of an individual to comply with instructions is in doubt, and family or friends are unable to ensure compliance, penicillamine should not be used.

Dose Regimen

No single dose regimen receives universal approval, but latterly most centres have tended to use lower doses, with more gradual increments than those of the original studies. A suggested treatment schedule is shown in Table 16.1. The rate of increase of the dose will depend on the individual patient. If the disease is very active and no side-effects are encountered, the dose may be increased 2 or 4 weekly to a total dose of 375 mg or 500 mg daily, and then held at this level for 4–6 weeks. If there is no response further increments in dose to a total of

750 mg (or at most 1000 mg) daily may be necessary. In the absence of side-effects, patients are encouraged to remain on treatment for at least 6 months and therapy is only discontinued if there is no subjective or objective improvement after several months at an adequate dose.

Table 16.1. Penicillamine therapy

1. Check FBC, platelets, urine, skin
2. Start 125 mg daily: 50 mg, 125 mg and 250 mg tablets available
    Specify dose precisely!
3. Increase dose by 125 mg every 4 weeks

Response:	Hold dose
	Cautiously reduce to maintenance dose
750 mg without response:	? Try increasing to 1000 mg daily
6 months' therapy with no response:	Review
	Stop therapy
	Try alternative after 'washout' period

4. Check blood, urine, skin 4 weekly throughout
5. Withhold/stop therapy if side-effects occur

Where minor side-effects occur, a more gradual increase in dose may be necessary. Occasionally treatment needs to be suspended for a period until minor adverse reactions settle, and then cautiously reintroduced.

After several months in remission the dose may be slowly reduced to a maintenance level which is continued indefinitely with 4-weekly monitoring.

At the time of initial prescription it should be stressed to the patient that response will be gradual and that penicillamine should supplement, and not replace, their anti-inflammatory medication.

Other Indications

It has been suggested that penicillamine is of benefit to patients with palindromic rheumatism, and those with rheumatoid vasculitis. Controlled studies are, however, not available in these conditions. Penicillamine has been shown to be of value in juvenile arthritis but not in seronegative spondylarthritides, progressive systemic sclerosis or chronic active hepatitis. A recent study suggests a possible role in primary biliary cirrhosis but this awaits confirmation.

Contraindications

Previous gold toxicity has been considered by some workers as an indication for caution since rashes and marrow aplasia may be more common, but this aspect has not been confirmed in other studies.

Pregnancy

Neonatal abnormalities (growth retardation, lax wrinkled skin and flexion contractures of hips and knees) have been reported in association with penicillamine treatment for rheumatoid arthritis during pregnancy. On the other hand, normal pregnancies have certainly occurred during penicillamine treatment in patients with Wilson's disease. Nevertheless, it is not considered justifiable to use a potentially hazardous drug during pregnancy in a disease such as rheumatoid arthritis which is not life threatening. A conservative approach is particularly indicated here since many patients experience a spontaneous remission while pregnant and only relapse postpartum. Penicillamine may be reintroduced after delivery and beneficial effect regained.

Genetic Predisposition

It has been suggested that patients with HLA DR3 are more likely to develop adverse reactions to penicillamine, and pretreatment tissue typing may be relevant in the future. However, this is expensive and time consuming and results from controlled prospective studies are required before firm conclusions can be drawn.

Interactions

Penicillamine has been shown to interact with iron and the two should not be given simultaneously. Penicillamine should be given as a single dose in the morning and, if necessary, iron as a single dose in the evening.

Toxicity

A wide variety of side-effects have been described in relation to penicillamine therapy. From a practical point of view they are discussed below systematically but there is also considerable variation in terms of severity—some adverse reactions are minor and require only symptomatic therapy while the occurrence of others makes withdrawal of penicillamine mandatory.

Bone Marrow

Platelets

Thrombocytopenia is the most prevalent blood dyscrasia and may occur at any stage of treatment and at any dose. There is usually a gradual decline in the platelet count which is reversible on withdrawal of penicillamine, and precipitous large falls are exceptional. Where there has been a fall in platelets and a prompt return to normal on cessation of therapy, a cautious second trial of penicillamine may occasionally be justified in patients who have responded. A second decline in platelets is an indication for final withdrawal of therapy. There has been controversy about the level of platelets which constitutes thrombocytopenia. In our laboratory the lower limit of normal is 150 000, and if the count is below this level therapy is suspended and the count checked. Technical problems do arise with clumping of platelets, which may give a spurious low count, but this should be evident if a blood film is inspected. Many patients with very active rheumatoid arthritis have a thrombocytosis, and a fall in platelets to within the normal range is associated with response to penicillamine therapy. This should not be considered an adverse reaction. This point is equally applicable to patients treated with gold and in both instances the practice of plotting sequential results gives an immediate visual check on progress.

Neutropaenia

This is uncommon and, as with thrombocytopenia, usually manifests as a gradual fall in white cell count which reverses on stopping penicillamine. Sudden large falls have been described but are exceedingly rare. Penicillamine should be withdrawn if there is a confirmed fall in the white cell count to below 4000.

Aplasia

Total aplasia has been recorded in the past when higher doses were used and where monitoring had failed. This remains a risk if patients default from follow up but continue to take their medication.

Kidney

Proteinuria

The incidence of proteinuria is difficult to gauge since definition and management vary amongst clinicians. Proteinuria may develop at any stage of treatment but commonly occurs between 6 and 18 months. The relevance of dose to the development of proteinuria is the subject of debate but no dose appears to be sufficiently low to be safe.

Penicillamine nephropathy has been studied both in patients with the nephrotic syndrome and in those with lesser degrees of proteinuria. Renal biopsy shows no change on light microscopy but electron dense deposits are seen on electron microscopy and are suggestive of the presence of immune complexes. These deposits occur in the same biopsies and with the same distribution as the immunofluorescent staining for IgG and C3, and there is some resemblance to idiopathic membranous nephropathy. Changes are similar to those described with gold nephropathy.

Proteinuria tends to diminish and eventually disappear on withdrawal of penicillamine, but there is evidence that the electron dense deposits persist even after protein is no longer detected in the urine. The significance of this is uncertain.

The degree of proteinuria which dictates cessation of therapy is yet another area of controversy. Our approach is to stop therapy if one plus or more is detected on dipstix in two urine samples and to arrange urine microscopy, culture, and 24-h quantitative protein measurement. In the absence of infection, therapy is withheld for as long as urinary protein exceeds 300 mg/24 h. When proteinuria disappears, a small dose of penicillamine is cautiously reintroduced. If proteinuria does not subside after several months off penicillamine, further investigation of the underlying cause is indicated. Where amyloidosis is shown on renal biopsy and the patient has benefited from penicillamine, therapy is restarted even in the face of nephrotic range proteinuria. In any other circumstances we consider proteinuria to be a contraindication to penicillamine therapy.

Haematuria

Cases of Goodpasture's syndrome have been reported during penicillamine therapy. Although this complication is rare, haematuria was the initial presenting feature and unexplained haematuria is thus considered an indication to stop treatment.

Skin

Rashes

Rashes occur at all stages of penicillamine therapy and have been observed at all doses. Early urticarial or morbilliform rashes settle rapidly on withdrawal of the drug, which, if the patient is agreeable, may then be reintroduced at a low dose. Later on in the course of treatment (most often between 6 and 12 months) irregular pruritic plaques may occur. These are characteristically seen mainly on the trunk and are scaly. They resolve very slowly after cessation of therapy and a further trial of penicillamine is probably contraindicated since this rash may represent a mild transient form of a potentially more serious rash, namely, pemphigus. Pemphigus foliaceus presents with scaling, crusting and blistering, but the blistering is not obvious as in pemphigus vulgaris. Pemphigus foliaceus is more commonly seen than pemphigus vulgaris and while it is not as aggressive, it may persist for several years despite systemic corticosteroid therapy.

Mouth Ulceration

Mouth ulcers indistinguishable from aphthous ulceration occur during penicillamine therapy and respond to reduction in dosage. In about 1% of patients it is necessary to discontinue therapy altogether because of recurrent painful ulceration.

Loss of Taste

Altered taste sensation has been emphasised in the past as a common side-effect of penicillamine. Nevertheless, we have encountered few patients who complain spontaneously of this symptom. Certainly it is seldom a management problem since normal taste tends to return over a period of weeks or months if patients are willing to continue therapy (and most patients will do so if given suitable reassurance).

Gastrointestinal

Nausea and vomiting can often be controlled by varying the dose regimen, but in a few individuals gastrointestinal upset is intolerable and penicillamine needs to be stopped. There is no convincing evidence that penicillamine causes peptic ulceration and although haematemeses have occurred in patients on this therapy, a causal relationship has not been established.

Rare Side-effects

Drug-induced SLE, Goodpasture's syndrome, polymyositis and myaesthenia have all been reported as adverse reactions to penicillamine therapy. While these syndromes are uncommon, it is essential to view unexplained symptoms and signs with suspicion and if necessary to withhold penicillamine until the situation has been clarified. Both SLE and myaesthenia improve on cessation of therapy but Goodpasture's syndrome has in most instances proved fatal.

A polyarthritis (ANA negative) has been described in patients with Wilson's disease, and some patients with rheumatoid arthritis complain of worsening joint symptoms following ingestion of penicillamine tablets.

Paradoxically, both alopecia (?ANA status) and hirsutism have been described on penicillamine therapy and mammary hyperplasia may rarely cause considerable discomfort. A recent report suggests that danazol may be of value in the latter syndrome.

Hepatic and pulmonary side-effects have occasionally been ascribed to penicillamine therapy but these claims have not yet been substantiated.

Conclusion

Penicillamine is a useful drug which may produce considerable symptomatic improvement in the rheumatoid patient, and in addition may slow progression of erosive disease. The danger of unsupervised therapy should the patient default from monitoring while still receiving repeat precription must be borne in mind. A register of patients started on penicillamine may help in this respect. The availability of 125 mg and 250 mg tablets is a further source of potential confusion, and meticulous attention to prescription by dose and not only by tablet number is necessary if this drug is to be used safely.

Further Reading

Bacon P, Tribe CR, Mackenzie JC et al. (1976) Penicillamine nephropathy in rheumatoid arthritis. Q J Med 180: 661–684

Day AT, Golding JR, Leek PN, Butterworth AD (1974) Penicillamine in rheumatoid disease: A long term study. Br Med J I: 180–184

Gibson T, Huskisson EC, Wojtulewski JA et al. (1976) Evidence that D-penicillamine alters the course of rheumatoid arthritis. Rheumatol Rehabil 15: 211–215

Hill FH (1980) Penicillamine in the treatment of rheumatoid arthritis. In Hill AGS (ed) Topical reviews in rheumatic disorders. Wright-PSG, Bristol London Boston, pp 78–109

Huskisson EC, Gibson JJ, Balme HW et al. (1974) Trial comparing D-penicillamine and gold in rheumatoid arthritis. Ann Rheum Dis 33: 532–535

Lyle WH (1979) Penicillamine. In: Huskisson E (ed) Clinics in rheumatic diseases. Saunders, Philadelphia London Toronto, pp 596–602

Marsden RA, Ryan TJ, Vanhegan RI et al. (1976) Pemphigus foliaceus induced by penicillamine. Br Med J II: 1423–1424

Multicentre Trial Group (1973) Controlled trial of D(-) penicillamine in severe rheumatoid arthritis. Lancet I: 275–280

Rosenbaum J, Katz WA, Schumacher HR (1980) Hepatotoxicity associated with the use of D-penicillamine in rheumatoid arthritis. Ann Rheum Dis 39: 152–154

17 Antimalarials and Other Second-Line Drugs

Antimalarials

History

The use of antimalarials in rheumatoid arthritis has had a chequered history since the publication of controlled studies in the 1950s.

Chemistry

Chloroquine (CQ) and hydroxychloroquine (HQ) are 4-aminoquinolines which are effective against the malarial parasite. Chloroquine phosphate is a white bitter powder which is soluble in water. The *d*-isomer is less toxic than the *l*-isomer. Hydroxychloroquine is formed by the hydroxylation of one of the *N*-ethyl substituents of chloroquine.

Pharmacology

Chloroquine and hydroxychloroquine are almost completely absorbed from the gastrointestinal tract and circulate in bound–free equilibrium with plasma proteins. At therapeutic concentrations approximately 55% is bound in the case of CQ. Excretion is mainly by the renal route, most of the drug appearing as desethylchloroquine or unchanged in urine. The renal excretory mechanism is enhanced by acidification and retarded by alkalinisation of the urine. Approximately 10% of the administered dose is excreted in the faeces and a substantial proportion of the remainder cannot be accounted for by either of these routes. It has been suggested that concentration and loss in hair and epidermal cells may be responsible for at least some of this discrepancy. Deposition in tissues rich in melanin and in parenchymatous organs is cumulative.

Rheumatological Indications

1. Rheumatoid Arthritis. Antimalarial enthusiasts advocate ready prescription of CQ and HCQ to patients with early rheumatoid arthritis, and continue this therapy indefinitely. At the other end of the spectrum are rheumatologists who refuse to use antimalarials at all. Discussion of the antimalarials should be placed in a "2nd line" context.

Much of the controversy centres on ocular toxicity, with contradictory reports in the literature. Certainly several studies have demonstrated that after a delay of several months both CQ and HCQ will produce symptomatic relief superior to placebo and lead to a fall in the erythrocyte sedimentation rate and in rheumatoid factor titres. While to date no radiological improvement has been documented, there is no doubt that these drugs produce significant benefit in many of the rheumatoid patients for whom they are prescribed. This benefit falls short of that seen in patients who respond to gold. The problem of toxicity is discussed in more detail below. Therapy should not be commenced without the cooperation of an ophthalmologist who will monitor the patient at least three times per year and, as always, with the informed consent of the patient. Blindness is an emotive topic and discussion of possible ocular toxicity needs careful handling. Many patients who remain unconcerned when bone marrow, skin or renal toxicity is discussed in relation to gold or penicillamine react dramatically and immediately to any mention of the possible visual adverse effects of chloroquine. Our policy is to explain that the drugs are safe in the first year if they are taken in the prescribed dose with appropriate ophthalmological monitoring. This should be undertaken before therapy is commenced and at 4-monthly intervals thereafter. We insist on a formal rheumatological review after 1 year to assess the advisability of further therapy. At this stage we emphasise that there may be a small risk of ocular toxicity and that regular monitoring remains mandatory. Patients who have shown significant improvement may elect to continue therapy. Alternatively treatment is discontinued for 3–6 months and if disease activity increases CQ or HCQ is reintroduced. As in other fields, the patient needs to understand the facts insofar as they are known since compliance is essential.

Both CQ and HCQ are effective and toxicity is reported with each. The recommended dose of chloroquine phosphate (Avloclor) is 250 mg daily and of hydroxychloroquine (Plaquenil) 200 mg b.d. Some authors have suggested a daily dose of 4 mg/kg CQ and 6 mg/kg HCQ, but the difficulty in dividing the tablets currently available makes calculating individual doses an unrewarding exercise. This is, however, of more importance if antimalarials are used in children (Laaksonen et al. 1974) since appropriate dose calculation is essential in paediatric practice. There is no evidence that monitoring serum concentrations is of value in predicting efficacy or toxicity.

2. Systemic Lupus Erythematosus. Antimalarials are thought to be of value in SLE, particularly for skin and joint manifestations, although there are no adequately controlled studies in this disease. In several small studies placebo was substituted for active antimalarial in SLE patients who had responded and almost all patients relapsed.

An initial dose larger than 250 mg CQ or 400 mg HCQ would allow equilibrium to be reached sooner than the 3–5 week period necessary when these conventional doses are employed and might produce earlier benefit. The higher initial dose, however, increases the incidence of unacceptable gastrointestinal side-effects and more patients withdraw from treatment. Since the role of antimalarials in rheumatology is not "life-saving", the slower, lower regimen is preferred. Dubois recommends constant, long-term use in SLE and has not observed retinal toxicity in his patients at doses given above. Monitoring in SLE, as in rheumatoid arthritis, needs to be conscientious.

3. Psoriatic Arthropathy. Cautious use in psoriatic arthropathy has been advocated after exfoliative dermatitis was described with quinacrine. This appears to be a rare event with CQ and HCQ but remains a risk which physician and patient should weigh up against anticipated benefit prior to initiating therapy.

No useful role for antimalarials has been demonstrated in progressive systemic sclerosis, Sjögren's syndrome, dermatomyositis, ankylosing spondylitis or other seronegative spondyloathropathies.

Toxicity

Many of the original reports on the toxicity of CQ and HQ refer to higher doses than those currently recommended. Accordingly, the literature needs to be closely scrutinised if a realistic assessment of dose-related toxicity is to be made. The eye is, of course, the major concern of the clinician, but many systems may be affected.

1. Ocular. Antimalarials may affect the cornea, lens, ocular smooth and striated muscle and retina. Corneal deposits are of no clinical importance other than in the production of symptoms which may mimic glaucoma, i.e. blurred vision and halos around lights. These deposits, and chloroquine-induced cataracts, are reversible on cessation of therapy and do not correlate with retinopathy. Transient presbyopia due to a direct effect on smooth muscle has been observed and on rare occasions abducent palsies may produce diplopia.

However, of all ocular adverse effects, retinopathy is the most worrying. CQ and HCQ have an affinity for pigmented areas and remain detectable there long after they have disappeared from non-pigmented tissue areas. They thus accumulate in organs rich in melanin such as the retina, where retinal photoreceptors are dependent on the integrity of retinal pigment epithelium. This pigment has an important nutritive function for rod and cone cells and participates in the restoration of photosensitive pigments. Interference with local metabolism may lead to significant visual loss. It has been suggested that sunlight and tobacco may potentiate the retinal toxicity of antimalarials. How can retinopathy be detected in time to prevent permanent visual loss? Were this question answered, use of CQ and HCQ would be considerably simpler. Rynes et al. (1979) have suggested monitoring:

1. Subjective assessment
2. Visual acuity
3. Fundoscopy—looking especially for granules or pigmentary changes in the retina
4. Red test object on visual fields
5. Slit lamp for corneal deposits
6. Accommodation
7. Electro-oculograms

Using this battery of tests they detected abnormalities in 3 of 99 patients treated with HCQ 400 mg daily for 13–68 months. All three patients with toxicity had rheumatoid arthritis although only 58 of the 99 patients were suffering from that disease. One of the three needed to stop therapy and this patient showed some improvement over the ensuing 2 years. Marks and Power (1979) followed up 222 patients (202 with rheumatoid arthritis and 20 with SLE) for periods of up to 8 years; 54 had been treated for less than 1 year. Ophthalmic assessment at 6-monthly intervals recorded visual acuity, slit lamp and fundal examination. Some patients also had visual field and colour vision testing, fluorescein angiography, and electroretinograms. Twenty-two of the 222 patients developed retinopathy, of whom five had the classical bull's eye lesion. Only one case showed progression of retinopathy, and in the other patients detection of the retinal abnormality was not necessarily associated with detectable visual loss. The occurrence of retinopathy was related to increasing age and to duration of therapy and dosage. Their recommendation was to use 250 mg CQ phosphate daily for 1 year and then to stop treatment. If the patient relapsed it was suggested that CQ be reintroduced, if possible on an alternate day or thrice weekly basis. Thus while the best mode of ophthalmological monitoring remains controversial, it would appear that low dose antimalarial therapy rarely produces significant ocular damage. Sun-glasses may exert a partial protective effect.

2. *Gastrointestinal.* Many patients complain of nausea or dyspepsia but gastrointestinal side-effects rarely force discontinuation of treatment. Lower bowel symptoms are usually transient.

3. *Skin and Hair.* Skin rashes on CQ usually take the form of lichenoid eruptions, but these are uncommon and reverse rapidly on withdrawal of treatment. Hyperpigmentation of the exposed skin in response to ultraviolet light may occur. A syndrome of localised cutaneous blue-black pigmentation involving the pretibial, palatal, facial and subungual areas has been reported. On biopsy heavy deposits of melanin and haemosiderin are seen. Bleaching of the hair and vitiligo may be associated with excessive dosage.

4. *Bone Marrow.* Aplastic anaemia may occur at high doses but has not yet been recorded at lower doses. Leucopenia and thrombocytopenia are rare and

usually reverse on withdrawal of treatment although fatal agranulocytosis has been described. "Toxic granulation" of leucocytes has been reported with CQ.

5. *Nervous System*. Although reported in association with CQ, convulsions have not been shown to be caused by this drug. Foetal ototoxicity may be produced by the use of this drug during pregnancy.

6. *Muscle*. Reversible myaesthenia may be produced by CQ. A vacuolar myopathy which produces a proximal symmetrical pattern may also occur. Muscle enzyme changes are absent and the syndrome will reverse on withdrawal of treatment.

7. *Heart*. Chloroquine has a negative chronotropic and inotropic effect and pre-existing conduction abnormalities are a contraindication to treatment with antimalarials. However, the commonly observed T-wave changes seen on ECG are not associated with the production of symptoms.

8. *Pregnancy*. Chromosome damage has been demonstrated and antirheumatic doses of CQ or HCQ are contraindicated in pregnancy.

Conclusion

It is valuable to keep a register of all patients who commence CQ or HCQ therapy to ensure adequate follow up. Even patients who are aware of the importance of regular monitoring may default and it is only too easy to lose track of such patients in a busy clinic.

Sulphasalazine

This drug is well established in the management of inflammatory bowel disease and it is ironic that it was introduced originally for the treatment of rheumatoid arthritis. Recent reports rediscovering the efficacy of this compound in patients with rheumatoid arthritis have emphasised that sulphasalazine does indeed have a "second line" effect. The dose recommended is in the range of 2–3 g daily. Gastrointestinal adverse reactions are common and there may also be an idiosyncratic reaction associated with skin rash, fever and leucopenia. Reversible sterility in male patients has been reported.

Levamisole

Although not available on prescription in the United Kingdom at present, this antihelminthic drug has been studied in patients with rheumatoid arthritis at doses ranging from 150 to 450 mg per week. It has been shown to produce a "second line" effect but only at the expense of considerable toxicity. In particular, leucopenia may occur.

Further Reading

Dubois EL (1978) Antimalarials in the management of discoid and systemic lupus erythematosus. Semin Arthritis Rheum 8: 35–51

Laaksonen A, Kosiahole V, Juva K (1974) Dosage of antimalarial drugs for children with juvenile rheumatoid arthritis and systemic lupus erythematosus. Scand J Rheumatol 3: 103–108

MacKenzie AH, Scherbel AL (1980) Chloroquine and hydroxychloroquine in rheumatological therapy. Saunders, Philadelphia London Toronto (Clin Rheum Dis, vol 10, pp 545–566)

Marks JS, Power BJ (1979) Is chloroquine obsolete in treatment of rheumatic disease? Lancet I: 371–373

Popert AJ, Meijers KAE, Sharp J, Bier F (1961) Chloroquine diphosphonate in rheumatoid arthritis. Ann Rheum Dis 20: 18–34

Rynes RI, Krohel G, Falbo A et al. (1979) Ophthalmologic safety of long term hydroxychloroquine treatment. Arthritis Rheum 22: 832–836

Scherbal AL, MacKenzie AH, Nousal JF, Atjidan M (1965) Ocular lesions in rheumatoid arthritis and related diseases with particular reference to retinopathy: a study of 741 patients treated with and without chloroquine drugs. N Engl J Med 273: 360–366

18 Corticosteroids

History

Corticosteroids have been used and abused in many conditions since their dramatic debut in 1948. This brief chapter will emphasise their toxicity, which may be considerable with prolonged use, while attempting to highlight indications for their prescription. Much of the relevant literature on the subject is more than 10 years old, and despite 30 years of use corticosteroids still exemplify the confusion and controversy which surround drug therapy in rheumatology.

Chemistry

The steroid nucleus consists of A, B and C (six carbon) rings and a D (five carbon) ring with a total of 17 carbon atoms. Substitution of hydrogen atoms attached to C10, 13 or 17 with side chains produces biologically important steroid compounds.

Steroids are classified as lipids because of their greater solubility in organic than in aqueous solvents, but all naturally occurring steroids are soluble in plasma at physiological concentrations. As the number of hydroxyl or carboxyl groups on the steroid nucleus increases, it becomes more soluble in water.

Endogenous corticosteroids are synthesised in the adrenal cortex, cholesterol being an essential intermediate in this process. They are secreted as they are produced and there is virtually no storage in the adrenal. Cortisol (hydrocortisone) is the major product of the adrenal cortex, which under basal conditions produces 12–30 mg/day with a diurnal variation. Control of secretion is regulated by ACTH (which is in turn controlled by corticotrophin-releasing factor produced by the hypothalamus) and by a negative feedback mechanism.

All currently used anti-inflammatory steroids are 17-hydroxy compounds. Substituents on the surface of the molecule interfere with its binding to plasma proteins and a high proportion of circulating steroid is thus kept in its active unbound form.

Pharmacological Actions

The pharmacological actions of corticosteroids are complex and diverse and only a brief outline of selective actions will be given.

Modifications of the structure of cortisone have increased the ratio of anti-inflammatory to sodium-retaining potency to the extent that electrolyte effects are usually not important even at high doses. However, the effect on carbohydrate and protein metabolism and on inflammation has remained quantitatively similar. Occasionally hypokalaemic alkalosis is observed but in general glucocorticoids have a low potency mineralocorticoid effect.

Carbohydrate Metabolism

Steroids increase hepatic gluconeogenesis in normal subjects, leading to a temporary rise in blood glucose. This is compensated by an increase in insulin secretion so that the initially impaired glucose tolerance is not a persistent feature. However, prolonged administration may exhaust pancreatic cells and lead to "steroid diabetes." In diabetic subjects there is a marked rise in blood glucose. Glucocorticoids also accelerate protein catabolism, induce resistance to glucose transport in muscle and inhibit glucose uptake by adipose tissue, skin fibroblasts and lymphoid tissue. If hyperglycaemia is sustained, there is a secondary increase in glycogen deposition in the liver. Prolonged steroid treatment will elevate glucagon concentration in the plasma.

Protein and Nucleic Acid Metabolism

Corticosteroids enhance total protein synthesis in the liver, but in most other sites, including muscle, bone and skin, and lymphoid, connective and adipose tissues, they lead to decreased synthesis and increased breakdown of protein. A state of negative nitrogen balance is thus induced. There is a diminished work capacity of striated muscle, but the mechanism of this is unclear.

Inhibition of DNA synthesis in liver muscle and kidney may partly account for growth retardation induced by steroid therapy. In addition growth hormone may be suppressed although attempts to overcome growth arrest by growth hormone replacement in steroid-treated children have been unsuccessful. Normal growth resumes on cessation of steroid therapy.

Lipid Metabolism

Prolonged steroid administration will lead to redistribution of body fat; the mechanism whereby fat is mobilised from the periphery and deposited centrally is unknown.

Corticosteroids alone have very little direct effect on lipid metabolism and produce no consistent change in serum lipid concentration. They do, however, facilitate catecholamine lipolysis of triglycerides in adipose tissue, leading to the release of free fatty acids and glycerol.

Water and Electrolytes

Glucocorticoids exert a weak mineralocorticoid effect on the distal tubule of the kidney, where they enhance sodium reabsorption from the tubular fluid and increase the excretion of potassium and hydrogen ions. Usually this produces no significant clinical effect but occasionally hypokalaemic alkalosis may result.

Inflammation and Wound Healing

In the presence of pharmacological doses of glucocorticoids, polymorphonuclear cell migration is suppressed and fewer of these cells are found at an inflammatory focus. There is an increase in the number of polymorphonuclear cells in circulation because of accelerated release from the bone marrow. Suppression of neutrophil phagocytosis is demonstrable in vitro but an in vivo effect has not yet been shown. Monocyte accumulation is inhibited, possibly as a result of delayed release from bone marrow, and monocytopenia is characteristic. Release of arachidonic acid from phospholipids is inhibited by corticosteroids and formation of prostaglandins and related compounds diminished. Liver lysosomes are stabilised by glucocorticoids but no similar effect has been observed on granulocyte lysosomal membranes.

While detailed mechanisms of effects on inflammation await further elucidation, a clear clinical message remains: the ability of glucocorticoids to suppress inflammation of varied aetiology is not without disadvantages. While this suppression may achieve a therapeutic goal, it is indiscriminate and may mask signs and symptoms of infection or of peptic ulcer perforation.

Another undesirable action of glucocorticoids is inhibition of fibroblast proliferation and of collagen formation by fibroblasts, leading to decreased tensile strength in wounds and a danger of dehiscence.

Blood, Lymphoid Tissue and Immune Responses

Haemoglobin, red cell count and polymorphonuclear leucocytes increase during glucocorticoid treatment, while numbers of lymphocytes, eosinophils, monocytes and basophils decrease.

Hypercorticism is characterised by a decreased mass of lymphoid tissue and by lymphocytopenia. The decrease in circulating lymphocytes may be due to sequestration from the blood as well as to lymphocytolysis, and T-lymphocytes are decreased proportionately more than B-lymphocytes.

The effect of glucocorticoids on humoral immunity is not clearly defined. Very large doses of methylprednisolone will produce a fall in concentrations of IgG in volunteers, but these subjects remain able to produce antibody normally in response to antigenic stimuli. Therapeutic use of steroid does not consistently affect the titres of circulating IgG or IgE or alter the metabolism of complement despite having an effect in "autoimmune" and allergic states.

It seems likely that steroids interfere not so much with cell-mediated immunity itself as with the subsequent events set in train by alteration in lymphocyte function. Reduction in the consequences of cell-mediated immunity occurs through suppression of inflammatory responses during delayed hypersensitivity reactions. For example, production of macrophage migration inhibitory factor (MIF) by lymphocytes is not affected, but the effect of MIF on macrophages is blocked.

The known pharmacological actions of glucocorticoids are thus diverse, yet their precise mode of action is still not fully understood. Advances in our knowledge of the cortisol receptor and its role in intracellular transport and the modulation of intranuclear control mechanisms offer hope for the future.

Absorption, Transport, Metabolism and Excretion

Prednisolone and other synthetic corticosteroids are well absorbed orally, while if a high concentration in body fluids is required rapidly, water-soluble steroid esters may be used for intravenous administration. Absorption is also effective, depending on the preparation, from synovial fluid and from skin. Most studies of steroid metabolism have been of cortisol and it is assumed that synthetic steroids will be broadly similar. Ninety per cent of cortisol is bound to two protein fractions, viz. to a corticosteroid-binding globulin (a glycoprotein) and to albumin. At low or normal concentrations most hormone is bound to globulin, which has high affinity but low total binding capacity. Both free and albumin-bound corticosteroid increase when the amount of corticosteroid is increased, while the globulin fraction is little changed. The plasma half-life of prednisolone is approximately 190 min, but the duration of action is much longer than plasma survival time because of distribution in body fluids.

A double bond is found in the C4,5 position and a ketone group at C3 in all active corticosteroids. The 4,5 double bond may be reduced at either hepatic or extrahepatic sites, yielding an inactive substance, while formation of tetrahydrocortisol by reduction of the 3-ketone to a 3-hydroxyl group apparently occurs only in the liver. Excretion is in the form of water-soluble esters or glucosides which are formed in the liver or kidney by coupling through the 3-hydroxyl group with sulphate or glucuronic acid.

Studies using labelled steroid have shown that most of the radioisotope is recovered in the urine within 72 h. It would appear that a higher proportion of synthetic corticosteroid is excreted unchanged in the urine, and less is conjugated with glucuronic acid than occurs with cortisol metabolism.

Therapeutic doses of phenobarbitone will produce measurable clinical deterioration in patients on prednisolone, probably by inducing hepatic metabolism and thus effectively reducing the steady state plasma level.

Rheumatological Indications

These drugs are in no way specific for rheumatological disorders. It is important that a decision to use steroids should not obscure the need for other measures, either initially or in the long term. We need to acknowledge that all too often in rheumatology steroids ameliorate the short-term problem without improving the long-term prognosis. They may be used either electively or, less commonly, in a life-threatening (or sight-threatening) situation. In both instances, treatment is palliative and empirical. Note that systemic corticosteroids are *not* indicated in (a) progressive systemic sclerosis or (b) osteoarthritis. Where used *electively*, careful consideration of indications and implications is mandatory. The clinician should ask the following questions before embarking on prolonged corticosteroid therapy:

1. What is the goal of steroid therapy in these patients?
2. Is there reliable evidence (in the literature) that steroids will achieve this goal?
3. Have all other simpler and less toxic alternatives been tried?
4. What is the smallest dose of steroid that is likely to be effective? Would intra-articular or topical therapy suffice?
5. Are there any specific contraindications or problems which will need additional safeguards, e.g. previous TB?
6. Is the patient aware of the benefits and risks of treatment and likely to co-operate?
7. Is alternate day therapy practicable?
8. How long will therapy need to be continued?

Indications for Elective Use

Rheumatoid Arthritis

There are two distinct approaches to the use of oral corticosteroids in rheumatoid arthritis: Pulse treatment with very high doses over a brief period in the context of sight- or life-threatening disease is being evaluated at the moment; otherwise the debate centres upon the use of long-term low dose corticosteroid therapy.

Most rheumatologists spend a considerable amount of time and effort in the thankless task of attempting to withdraw corticosteroids in patients who have found this regimen to be destructive and ineffective in the long term. This makes it so much more important that we avoid the mistakes of the past and eschew meddlesome interference. Corticosteroids should only very rarely be considered for the treatment of patients with rheumatoid arthritis and then only after all other possible avenues have been explored. In the dose which may be effective, toxicity is prohibitive, and the dose which may be safe is ineffective. Without doubt, corticosteroids fall into the category of "third line" drugs.

If the decision is made to embark upon long-term low dose corticosteroid therapy then prednisolone (1 mg tablets) is the drug of choice; doses in the range of 5–7.5 mg must not be exceeded. Treatment should be started with a small dose, e.g. 4 or 5 mg, and gradually be increased to 7.5 mg only if absolutely necessary.

Steroids should be discontinued if prompt symptomatic relief is not obtained. Regimens which initially employ high doses and which then cut back over days or weeks are not recommended. At high doses patients may experience complete pain relief but their expectation for the future will be unrealistic; the high dose cannot be continued indefinitely because of the danger of cumulative toxicity, and over a period of years patients stabilised on a particular dose appear to require an increased amount of corticosteroid to achieve equivalent benefit. Early in steroid therapy there may be a feeling of well-being or even euphoria; the ESR may fall in the first few months and the haemoglobin rise. These benefits are lost once therapy continues beyond a few months, and multicentre studies have demonstrated no benefit of hydrocortisone over aspirin over 2 or 3 years. There is certainly no evidence that steroids will retard the progression of rheumatoid disease; indeed, it has been suggested that this therapy may accelerate erosive changes and be implicated in the development of rheumatoid vasculitis. These two suggestions remain unproven but are of concern to the clinician. It is now established that even very low doses on a continuous basis will accelerate osteopenia.

Alternate day therapy should be attempted to minimise adrenal suppression. If an alternate day regimen is not possible, a single daily dose taken in the morning should be tried.

Systemic Lupus Erythematosus

The diagnosis of SLE does not in itself imply that corticosteroid therapy will be necessary. Many patients with SLE are successfully managed by simple measures alone (see Chap. 12), and others need steroids for only short spells.

Again, in most instances there should be time for a comprehensive assessment of all systems and an unhurried appraisal of anticipated benefits and risks. Although steroids are often prescribed for renal and cerebral lupus, there may be a case for conservative management. Dramatic benefit from corticosteroids may be observed in haemolytic anaemia, but manifestations such as polyserositis, polyarthritis (which is conspicuously non-destructive in the great majority of instances) and skin involvement do not usually require corticosteroids and may be managed by more simple general measures.

Polymyositis and Dermatomyositis

Prednisolone is the drug of choice in these conditions and should be tried alone for a reasonable period before considering additional cytotoxic therapy. When used electively, careful titration of dose in accordance with symptoms and signs often allows adjustment to a minimal dose with gratifying results.

Mixed Connective Tissue Disease

This syndrome is steroid sensitive but it is often worthwhile trying a single non-steroidal drug of the patient's own choice in the first instance.

Polymyalgia Rheumatica

In the absence of eye symptoms or signs a modest dose of prednisolone (less than 10 mg using 1 mg tablets, which allow minor dose adjustment) may produce a gratifying response. In fact failure of response should throw doubt upon the original diagnosis.

Polyarteritis Nodosa

This very rare disease provides an indication for the exhibition of corticosteroids despite the absence of controlled data on the subject.

Wegener's Granulomatosis

For many years this horrific disease was treated by corticosteroids alone with indifferent results. Only very recently have well-controlled long-term studies been conducted and these leave no doubt that the optimum treatment is cyclophosphamide with or without the addition of prednisolone. These carefully conducted studies have demonstrated a dramatic improvement in the prognosis of this disease when it is recognised early and treated properly.

Eosinophilic Fasciitis

As is the case with mixed connective tissue disease, this syndrome is steroid responsive but there is a case to be made for attempting to control the symptoms with a non-steroidal drug in the first instance.

Imperative Indications

On rare occasions it may be necessary to commence steroids while still investigating and assessing a patient:

1. *Giant cell arteritis* (see Chap. 10): Where temporal arteritis is suspected, high dose (>60 mg/day) steroid therapy should be started immediately, even while a biopsy is being arranged or while the histology is awaited.
2. *Polymyositis with weakness of respiratory muscles* (see Chap. 11): Prompt in-patient administration of large doses of steroid will be required in this unusual but life-threatening circumstance.
3. *Fulminating systemic lupus erythematosus* (see Chap. 12): It is vital that co-existent infection is actively sought and vigorously treated if large dose steroid is used in this situation.
4. *Iridocyclitis uncontrolled by topical therapy* (see Chap. 13)

Preparations

There is abundant literature commenting on the advantages and disadvantages of ACTH versus oral steroid therapy but a dearth of properly controlled studies. In general ACTH appears to confer no additional therapeutic benefit but does avoid adrenal suppression and possibly growth retardation in children. Hypertension and hypokalaemia may be more of a problem with ACTH and multiple injections are inconvenient in the long-term management of rheumatological disorders. On the other hand osteopenia may be less of a problem. The pigmentation of the patient receiving ACTH is due to the MSH sequence within the ACTH molecule.

The majority of patients who require protracted corticosteroid therapy are best managed with an oral preparation. Choice of this preparation is a controversial issue and while it is generally accepted that none of the newer synthetic oral corticosteroids is any better than prednisolone there is no firm evidence of this. Nevertheless, in our current state of knowledge prednisolone is the steroid of choice—it is inexpensive, is available in 1 mg and 5 mg tablets which allow flexibility and gradual dose adjustments, and has an intermediate duration of action. The latter property is necessary if a rational attempt at alternate day therapy is to be made (Table 18.1).

Table 18.1. Duration of action of glucocorticoids

Short-acting	Cortisol (hydrocortisone)
	Cortisone
Intermediate-acting	Prednisone
	Prednisolone
	Triamcinolone
Long-acting	Dexamethasone

It is sensible to become familiar with the potency of corticosteroid preparations: equivalent doses of oral steroids are shown in Table 18.2. Conversion from more potent preparations to prednisolone prior to attempted steroid withdrawal will facilitate small dose reductions and allow a flexible regimen.

Table 18.2. Equivalent doses of commonly used gluco-corticoids

Glucocorticoid	Dose (mg)
Cortisol (hydrocortisone)	20
Cortisone	25
Prednisolone	5
Prednisone	5
Triamcinolone	4
Methylprednisolone	4
Dexamethasone	0.75
Betamethasone	0.75

Effective steroid drugs require the presence of a hydroxyl group at carbon 11. Thus the 11-keto compounds cortisone and prednisone lack glucocorticoid activity until converted to hydrocortisone and prednisolone by the liver. In the presence of hepatic disease either hydrocortisone or prednisolone should be employed.

Aborption of prednisolone from plain and enteric-coated preparations is equal, although enteric-coated therapy produces a lower peak plasma level which occurs later. Bioavailability is similar, but reduction in gastrointestinal intolerance with the enteric-coated form has not been conclusively demonstrated.

The more potent preparations (dexamethasone, betamethasone) may find particular application in emergency situations such as cerebral oedema or rheumatic fever bordering on heart failure.

Toxicity

Corticosteroid toxicity remains a major worry for the prescribing physician and the list of side-effects in Table 18.3 is familiar but formidable. Prolonged therapy is more likely to be hazardous and the risk increases with increasing dose of steroid. It is noteworthy that studies of toxicity conducted in patients with respiratory disease are not necessarily applicable to rheumatic disorders. A detailed review of the consequences of corticosteroid therapy has been compiled by David et al. (1970) Unfortunately it is not possible to predict which patients will be particularly susceptible to adverse reactions, although a low serum albumin has been suggested as a factor which will predispose to the development of toxicity at lower than anticipated doses.

Table 18.3. Side-effects of glucocorticoid therapy

Endocrine	Suppression of HPA axis
	Growth retardation
	Menstrual irregularity
Metabolic	Glucose intolerance
	Redistribution of lipid
	(centripetal obesity)
	Hepatic microsomal enzyme induction
	Protein catabolism
Skin/subcutaneous tissue	Impaired wound healing
	Purpura, ecchymosis
	Plethora, striae, acne, hirsutism
	Moon face, buffalo hump, oedema
Musculoskeletal	Osteopenia, vertebral compression and long bone fractures, aseptic necrosis, myopathy
Gastrointestinal	Increased appetite, enhanced complications of peptic ulceration, e.g. perforation/haemorrhage, pancreatitis
Fluid balance	Oedema, hypertension
	Hypokalaemic acidosis
CNS and eye	Psychiatric disorders
	Intracranial hypertension
	Posterior subcapsular cataracts
	Glaucoma
Vascular	? Vasculitis
	Thromboembolism
	Accelerated atherosclerosis
Defence mechanisms	Increased risk of infection
	Masking of signs of infection
Pregnancy	? Increased liability to abortion

The smallest effective dose should be used for as short a time as possible if toxicity is to be minimised. While alternate day therapy or ACTH may protect the HPA axis and diminish growth retardation, other adverse effects may be unavoidable. Corticosteroids and ACTH are, therefore, dangerous drugs and the practicability of dose reduction should be regularly reviewed. Constant vigilance for the development of side-effects is mandatory and when these occur treatment should be prompt, lest major morbidity overshadows therapeutic benefit.

Steroid-Induced Diabetes

Steroid-induced diabetes is usually mild and easily controlled; these patients are not prone to ketoacidosis and hyperglycaemia reverses on cessation of steroids.

Steroid-Induced Osteopenia

Steroid-induced osteopenia is more common in the female and in children and affects the ribs and the vertebral bodies most severely. The precise role of calcium, vitamin D, oestrogen and more recent additions to the list of proposed remedies, including calcitonin, fluoride, the diphosphonates and hydroxyapatite, awaits definition.

Peptic Ulceration

It may be debated whether or not corticosteroids produce peptic ulceration but there is no doubt that they predispose to, and enhance the severity of, the complications of peptic ulceration, including perforation and haemorrhage. Thus it is important to bear this possibility in mind during treatment with these hormones. It is being suggested at the moment that H_2 receptor blocking drugs such as cimetidine may have a prophylactic role in protection from "stress ulceration" and this possibility may be explored in the context of corticosteroid-induced peptic ulceration.

Susceptibility to Infection

Not only are patients receiving corticosteroids more likely to develop infections, but the usual clinical signs of an inflammatory response which so often give the clue to their presence are suppressed. Unusual "opportunistic" organisms are the rule rather than the exception, and a high index of suspicion is appropriate.

Steroid Myopathy

This is usually seen at high dose and does not seem to be a function of cumulative low dose regimens. The onset is insidious and the most difficult clinical situation is in the patient who is receiving corticosteroid therapy for polymyositis. Differentiation is vital since in the one instance management is to increase and in the other to reduce the dose. In steroid myopathy serum enzymes and potassium are normal, and biopsy and EMG are usually not distinctively abnormal as they are in the exacerbation of the inflammatory disease. Urinary creatinine concentrations may be increased in both. An acute hydrocortisone myopathy has been described in young asthmatics receiving large doses of hydrocortisone over a short period but this has not yet been recorded in a rheumatological context. Pathologically the muscle fibres show vacuolar changes. It has been suggested that fluorodinated derivatives such as triamcinolone are particularly liable to be associated with myopathy.

Ocular Complications

These need special vigilance. A rise in intraocular pressure occurs frequently in patients treated with corticosteroid, but glaucoma is rare. Posterior subcapsular cataract is more common but usually occurs only after long-term treatment. Perhaps the most important adverse effect of corticosteroid upon the eye is predisposition to infection.

Collagen Changes

There is no doubt that corticosteroids affect adversely the state of the intercellular matrix or ground substance. McConkey's sign refers to the association between skin thinning and vertebral osteopenia, both of which may occur together in the absence of corticosteroid therapy. However, both tend to be more common and more severe in patients receiving long-term steroids. Increased skin fragility, subcutaneous atrophy, delayed wound healing, myopathy and osteopenia may all in part owe their origin to corticosteroid-induced negative nitrogen balance. There is also an interesting change in calcium distribution. In those patients with the most severe osteopenia there is often pronounced vascular calcification (Monckeburg's sclerosis) in the large and middle sized vessels. The basis of this redistribution and whether or not corticosteroids play a role in its production is not yet clear.

Other Complications

There are many other adverse effects of corticosteroid therapy (Table 18.3). Two additional and somewhat surprising toxic effects are true allergy, which is very rare, and anaphylaxis, which has only been documented with ACTH.

Conclusion

Use of Long-Term Corticosteroids

1. Use the smallest possible dose
2. Ensure that the patient and the family understand the risk/benefit ratio, the reason for starting and the recommended regimen.
3. Provide documentation (a cardboard "steroid" card)
4. Consider the possibility of alternate day therapy
5. Establish a therapeutic goal
6. If the goal is not attained within a short time (e.g., 3–4 weeks at most), *abandon*
7. Ensure regular follow up and attempt to reduce/withdraw at every visit
8. Side-effects become more of a problem with prolonged treatment; in particular, check the blood pressure, urine, bone and eyes

Always aim to discontinue corticosteroids as soon as possible.

Corticosteroid Withdrawal

1. Explanation, communication and observation are vital
2. Begin gradually (e.g. 10% of the dose per week)
3. Consider changing to alternate day regimen
4. Monitor closely the underlying disease; patients will often feel poorly (psychological dependence) when their underlying disease is either unaltered or even improving
5. Deterioration may represent features inherent in corticosteroid withdrawal (e.g. fever, myalgia, arthralgia, malaise, gastrointestinal upset and vomiting) rather than "flare-up" of the underlying arthritis. This should be discussed with the patient in advance
6. Be prepared to increase dose during intercurrent disease

Note: Abnormal short synacthen test indicating suppression of the HPA axis does not constitute a contraindication to withdrawal. Awareness of the enhanced danger of stress or infection is equally important whether or not there is evidence of suppression. The HPA axis may take 1–3 years to recover.

Neither corticosteroid prescription nor corticosteroid withdrawal should be undertaken lightly.

Further Reading

Askeri M, Vigios PJ Jr, Moskowitz RW (1976) Steroid myopathy in connective tissue diseases. Am J Med 61: 485–492

Bacon PA, Myles AB, Berntwell CG, Daly JR, Savage O (1966) Corticosteroid withdrawal in rheumatoid arthritis. Lancet II: 935–937

Castles JJ (1979) Clinical pharmacology of glucocorticoids. In: Hollander JL, McCarty DJ Jr (eds) Arthritis and allied conditions, 9th edn. Lea and Febiger, Philadelphia

David DS, Grieco MH, Cushman P (1970) Adrenal glucocorticoids after twenty years. A review of their clinical relevant consequences. J Chronic Dis 22: 637–711

Fauci AS, Dale DC, Barlow JE (1976) Glucocorticosteroid therapy; mechanisms of action and clinical considerations. Ann Intern Med 84: 304–315

Haynes RC, Murad F (1980) Adrenocorticotrophic hormone, adrenocortical steroids and their synthetic analogues. In: Goodman WS, Gillman AC (eds) The pharmacological basis of therapeutics, 6th edn. Macmillan, New York, pp 1466–1496

Jasani MK, Boyle JA, Dick WC, Williamson J, Taylor AK, Buchanan WW (1968) Corticosteroid induced H.P.A. axis suppression. Ann Rheum Dis 27: 352–359

Koch-Weser J, Buyny RL (1976) Withdrawal from glucocorticoid therapy. N Engl J Med 295: 30–32

McConkey B, Davies P, Crockson RA. Crockson AP (1979) Effects of gold, dapsone and prednisolone on serum C-reactive protein, haptoglobin and the erythrocyte sedimentation rate in rheumatoid arthritis. Ann Rheum Dis 38: 141–144

Nuki G, Jasani MK, Downie WW, Whaley K, Dick WC, Williamson J, Paterson RWW, Boyle C, Buchanan WW (1970) Clinicopharmacological studies on depot tetracosactrin in patients with rheumatoid arthritis. Pharm Clin 2: 99–108

Williamson J, Paterson RWW, McGavin DDM et al. (1969) Posterior subcapsular cataracts and glaucoma associated with long term oral corticosteroid therapy. Br J Ophthalmol 53: 361–372
Zutschi DW, Friedman M, Ansell BM (1971) Corticotrophin therapy in juvenile chronic polyarthritis (Still's disease) and effect on growth. Arch Dis Child 46: 584–593

19 Cytotoxic Drugs

Introduction

Much thought is necessary before a cytotoxic drug is prescribed in patients suffering from rheumatic disorders. These drugs pose dual problems when used in chronic disease: firstly, there is the danger of immediate toxicity (which is, of course, true of most drugs), and secondly there is the risk of a long-term effect on spermatogenesis and oogenesis and the possibility of predisposition to lymphoreticular and solid tissue neoplasms. The potential hazards must be carefully weighed against anticipated benefit, and antimitotic drugs should only be used after a careful trial of less toxic alternatives. Discussion with the patient and family is always essential. These drugs should be viewed in a "3rd" or even "4th line" context.

Several cytotoxic drugs have been tried in rheumatology: this discussion will, however, be limited to azathioprine, cyclophosphamide and methotrexate (Table 19.1).

Table 19.1.

Drug	Watchpoints
All cytotoxics	FBC
	Reproductive function
Azathioprine	Renal function—adjust dose
	Concurrent allopurinol therapy
Cyclophosphamide	Renal function—adjust dose
	Urinary output
	Frequency of bladder voiding
	Concurrent allopurinol therapy
Methotrexate	Presence of ascites/pleural effusion
	Concurrent drugs which are protein bound
	Hepatic function

Azathioprine

History

Azathioprine has only been introduced into rheumatological practice relatively recently, although the study of purine analogues dates back to 1942.

Chemistry

Azathioprine is an antimetabolite derived from 6-mercaptopurine by the addition of a substituted imidazole group. In vivo, azathioprine is metabolised to 6-mercaptopurine (which is an analogue of hypoxanthine), but the imidazole group alters transport and tissue selectivity, and thus confers different properties on the two drugs. If given together, however, their immunosuppressive effect is diminished.

Mechanism of Action

Azathioprine is a non-specific agent which affects cells at all stages of the maturation cycle. As is the case with other purine analogues, the precise mechanism which produces cell death is not known.

Absorption, Distribution, Metabolism and Excretion

Oral azathioprine is readily absorbed and cleared from the blood by degradation, tissue uptake and urinary excretion. Patients with reduced creatinine clearance will thus need dose reduction. Inhibition of xanthine oxidase impairs the conversion of azathioprine to 6-thiouric acid; therefore if allopurinol is administered concurrently the dose of azathioprine should be reduced (to approximately 25% of the normal dose).

Indications

1. Rheumatoid Arthritis. In studies of the treatment of active rheumatoid arthritis, doses ranging from 1.3 to 2.1 mg/kg/day have been shown to be as effective as gold or chloroquine, and doses of 2.5 mg/kg/day as effective as penicillamine. It has been demonstrated that azathioprine may possess an anti-inflammatory effect but is not an immunosuppressant at the doses prescribed conventionally.

2. SLE. The use of azathioprine in lupus nephritis remains experimental.

3. Polymyositis. Azathioprine may have a steroid-sparing effect in severe disease.

Monitoring

Check the full blood count weekly during the first 8 weeks of therapy or after dose increments. In the long-term 4-weekly blood checks will be necessary.

Preparations

Fifty-milligram tablets and 50-mg vials for injection are available. To some extent single tablet size limits fine oral dose adjustments.

Toxicity

1. Bone Marrow Depression. Leucopenia occurs more commonly than thrombocytopenia or anaemia, and occasionally a sudden fall in the white cell count is seen. Dose adjustment may solve the problem but sudden falls should lead to treatment withdrawal.

2. Predisposition to Infection. Life-threatening infections may arise during cytotoxic therapy and are particularly likely to be due to opportunistic infections. Be alert for these.

3. Toxic Hepatitis and Biliary Stasis. Azathioprine should be withheld in the presence of an elevated bilirubin level.

4. Others. Stomatitis, skin rash, alopecia, fever and gastrointestinal upset occur during azathioprine therapy. Reduction of dose may be sufficient to control these side-effects.

Conclusion

If well monitored, azathioprine therapy may occasionally be justified in aggressive rheumatological disease. Prescription without adequate supervision is unacceptable. Adjust the dose appropriately in the presence of renal impairment or concurrent allopurinol therapy.

Cyclophosphamide

History

Nitrogen mustards were first synthesised more than a century ago, and their potential toxicity was widely recognised during the 1914–1918 war. Cyclophosphamide was developed relatively recently in an attempt to achieve greater selectivity for neoplastic cells and controlled studies in malignancy were carried out during the 1960s.

Chemistry

A cyclic phosphamide group has replaced the *N*-methyl of the reference mustard, viz. mechlorethamine. The resulting alkylating compound is relatively inert and is stable in aqueous solution.

Pharmacological Actions

Cyclophosphamide acts on cells throughout the cell cycle, but has a greater effect during the S phase. There is a cytotoxic action on all rapidly proliferating tissues, which produces both therapeutic effect and unwanted toxicity. Non- dividing cells may be alkylated but in the absence of a stimulus to divide, the DNA repair enzymes of the cell appear to provide sufficient protection.

Absorption, Distribution, Metabolism and Excretion

Cyclophosphamide is well absorbed orally and has a plasma half-life of approximately 6–7 h. Prior treatment with allopurinol prolongs the half-life although the mechanism of this action is unclear.

Metabolism by hepatic microsomal enzymes yields a number of active metabolites. A secondary reaction in the liver produces inactive substances and may be protective to hepatic cells. Excretion is mainly renal although after oral administration some unchanged drug may be found in the stool.

Rheumatological Indications

1. Systemic Vasculitis. Vasculitis is rare but probably represents the best established rheumatological indication for cyclophosphamide therapy. Fauci et al. (1978) used 2 mg/kg in 16 patients with systemic vasculitis and achieved remission and reduction of steroid in all (although very little is said about toxicity encountered in achieving this remission).

2. Rheumatoid Arthritis. Cyclophosphamide may produce an effect in rheumatoid arthritis comparable to that of gold. However, the possible toxicity, especially in the long-term, limits its use in all but the most exceptional cases. The dose appropriate for rheumatoid arthritis is controversial. Townes et al. (1976) suggest 1.8 mg/kg/day. However, in practice tablets come in 50 mg strength and in adults 75 mg–100 mg/day may be used initially, increasing to 150 mg/day.

3. Systemic Lupus Erythematosus. The place of cyclophosphamide in the treatment of lupus nephritis is not adequately established. Alone there is no benefit; in conjunction with prednisolone there may be marginal benefit, but no controlled data exist.

Preparations

Fifty-milligram tablets and vials for injection of 100 mg, 200 mg and 500 mg are available. Again, this means that fine adjustments of oral therapy are not feasible.

Toxicity

The use of cyclophosphamide is associated with considerable toxicity which needs to be weighed against anticipated benefit.

1. Marrow Depression. Lymphocytes are more susceptible to damage than granulocytes, red cell precursors or megakaryocytes. Regular (weekly initially and 4-weekly long-term) blood counts are mandatory.

2. Urinary Collecting System. Damage to transitional epithelial cells of the urinary collecting system has been attributed to chemical irritation from metabolites of cyclophosphamide. Dysuria or haematuria occurs in 5%–10% of patients, and when either is detected, cyclophosphamide therapy should be stopped immediately. If therapy is continued in the face of haemorrhagic cystitis, intractable haemorrhage, chronic cystitis and bladder carcinoma may occur. Damage to the epithelium appears to be enhanced by high concentrations of metabolites in contact with the bladder for long periods of time. Thus high fluid intake and frequent voiding of urine are recommended during cyclophosphamide therapy.

3. Damage to Germinal Epithelium; Teratogenic and Carcinogenic Effects. Azoospermia with normal potency occurs in almost all males treated with high dose cyclophosphamide. Amenorrhoea is reported in some premenopausal females but is by no means invariable. Permanent sterility may result if cyclophosphamide is used in children. An increased risk of malignancy, especially non-Hodgkin's lymphoma, has been demonstrated in patients who receive cyclophosphamide for 3 months or more, and teratogenecity precludes use in pregnancy.

4. Nausea and Vomiting. Gastrointestinal upset is common but seldom necessitates withdrawal of therapy. This is presumed to be a central effect on the nervous system but is ill understood.

5. Alopecia. Hair follicles are especially vulnerable to the damaging effects which cyclophosphamide exerts on epithelial tissues. Alopecia is dose related and is reversible. Various authors have commented that this side-effect is well tolerated if the drug is effective, but warning of the likely development of alopecia seems advisable.

6. Miscellaneous. Mucosal ulceration, transverse ridging of the nails, increased skin pigmentation, pulmonary fibrosis, myocardial and hepatic toxicity and convulsions have all been reported in patients on cyclophosphamide.

7. Infection. Opportunistic infection is an ever-present risk.

Conclusion

In rare instances cyclophosphamide may prove life-saving. When life is not threatened, it should be reserved for severe disease which has failed to respond to an adequate trial of less toxic alternatives. Monitoring should be meticulous and failure to respond to a reasonable dose after 4–6 months should lead to withdrawal of therapy. Ensure that a high urinary output is maintained, and adjust the dose if renal function is impaired.

Methotrexate

Introduction

The therapeutic potential of methotrexate has been recognised for a quarter of a century and its clinical applications have been diverse. It is perhaps most widely used in rheumatology in the treatment of psoriasis and psoriatic arthropathy. While the advent of PUVA may alter the indications for methotrexate, it is likely to maintain a role in severe disease in the foreseeable future.

Pharmacological Actions

Methotrexate is a folate antagonist which inhibits the formation of tetrahydrofolic acid. The synthesis of DNA is affected and tissues with a high degree of mitotic activity are most sensitive to the folate antagonists. Cells are killed during the S phase of the cell cycle and the drug seems more effective during the logarithmic than during the plateau phase of growth. However, RNA and protein synthesis are also inhibited by methotrexate, which slows the entry of cells into the S phase, and to some extent the cytotoxic reaction may be self-limiting.

Absorption Rate and Excretion

Methotrexate is readily absorbed from the gastrointestinal tract and from parenteral sites. Approximately 50% is bound to plasma protein. The plasma concentration is directly proportional to the administered dose and other protein-bound drugs such as sulphonamides or salicylates may displace methotrexate. After intravenous therapy handling of the drug is triphasic. The first phase leads to distribution of methotrexate into body fluids while the second phase involves clearance by the kidney. In the third phase distribution into the pleural or pericardial cavities may occur, in which case an effusion may act as a reservoir and delayed release of the drug may contribute to toxicity.

Renal excretion is by glomerular filtration and tubular secretion. Most of a large dose and about 50% of a small dose is excreted unchanged in the urine and drugs which compete for tubular secretion may affect the rate of excretion. With very high doses a potentially nephrotoxic metabolite may be found.

Rheumatological Indications

1. Psoriatic Arthropathy. Methotrexate may be indicated in severe psoriatic arthropathy which has not responded to anti-inflammatory drugs. Psoriasis and associated arthritis will not clear completely during methotrexate therapy, but may improve to the extent that topical treatment and NSAIDs will give adequate control. Oral or parenteral therapy should be given once a week, rather than as a small daily dose.

2. Polymyositis. Methotrexate may have a steroid-sparing effect in polymyositis.

Preparations

Tablets of 2.5 mg and 10 mg and ampoules of 2.5 mg, 5 mg, 25 mg and 50 mg are available. The injectible forms are colour coded according to strength.

Toxicity

Toxicity is increased in patients on daily regimens and in malnourished or alcoholic individuals. All tissues with high mitotic activity are vulnerable.

1. Gastrointestinal. Ulcerative stomatitis and diarrhoea occur fairly frequently and often require cessation of therapy. Haemorrhagic enteritis and intestinal perforation are rare.

2. Hepatic. Hepatic toxicity may be diminished by using weekly i.v. therapy rather than a continuous low dose oral regimen. Liver function tests are not a good indication of liver damage and yearly liver biopsy during therapy has been recommended. Approximately 3% of psoriatic patients followed prospectively have developed cirrhosis.

3. Bone Marrow. Regular (weekly prior to i.v.) blood checks are necessary since methotrexate may produce bone marrow suppression.

4. Skin and Hair. Alopecia is temporary and dermatitis unusual.

5. Nephrotoxicity. This may be diminished by maintaining a high urinary output.

6. Reproductive Function. Defective oogenesis and spermatogenesis as well as increased spontaneous abortion and teratogenesis have been reported. Thus this therapy should not be used in child-bearing years without appropriate contraception (which should be continued for at least 3 months after cessation of methotrexate).

Conclusion

When using methotrexate it is important to maintain a good alkaline urinary output. Be careful if there is ascites or a pleural effusion. Knowledge of the pharmacokinetics is particularly important here and oncology colleagues should be consulted if in doubt. This is not a drug for the enthusiastic amateur.

Further Reading

Barnes CG, Lovatt GE (1982) Therapeutic workshop. Ann Rheum Dis 41[Suppl]: 1–60

Black RL, O'Brien WM, van Scott EJ, Auerback R, Eisen AZ, Burn JJ (1964) Methotrexate therapy in psoriatic arthritis. JAMA 189: 743

Cooperating Clinics of the American Rheumatism Association (1970) A controlled trial of cyclophosphamide in rheumatoid arthritis. N Engl J Med 283: 883–889

Donadio JV, Holley KE, Ferguson RH, Ilstrup DM (1976) Progressive lupus glomerulonephritis. Treatment with prednisone and combined prednisone and cyclophosphamide. Mayo Clin Proc 51: 484

Donadio JV, Holley KE, Wagner RD, Ferguson RH, McDuffie FC (1977) Further observations on the treatment of lupus nephritis with prednisone and combined prednisone and azathioprine. Arthritis Rheum 20: 685–692

Dwosh IL, Stein HB, Urowitz MB, Smythe HA, Hunter T, Ogryzlo MA (1977) Azathioprine in the treatment of rheumatoid arthritis; comparison with gold and chloroquine. Arthritis Rheum 20: 685–692

Fauci AS, Haynes BF, Katz P (1978) The sprectrum of vasculitis: clinical, pathologic, immunologic and therapeutic considerations. Ann Intern Med 89(1): 660–676

Kinlen LJ, Sheil AGR, Peto J, Doll R (1979) Collaborative United Kingdom–Australasian study of cancer in patients treated with immunosuppressive drugs. Br Med J II: 1461–1466

Schein PS, Winokier SH (1975) Immunosuppressive and cytotoxic chemotherapy: long-term complications. Ann Intern Med 82: 84–95

Steinberg AD, Kaltreich HB et al. (1971) Cyclophosphamide in lupus nephritis: A controlled trial. Ann Intern Med 75: 165

Townes AS, Sowa JM, Shulman LE (1976) Controlled trial of cyclophosphamide in rheumatoid arthritis. Arthritis Rheum 19: 563–573

Van Scott EJ, Auerbach R, Weinstein GD (1964) Parenteral methotrexate in psoriasis. Arch Dermatol 89: 550–556

Weinstein GD (1977) Methotrexate. Ann Intern Med 86: 199–204

Weinstein GD, Frost P (1971) Methotrexate for psoriasis. A new therapeutic schedule. Arch Dermatol 103: 33

Williams HJ, Reading JC, Ward JR, O'Brien WM (1980) Comparison of high and low dose cyclophosphamide therapy in rheumatoid arthritis. Arthritis Rheum 23: 521–527

20 Surgery

Introduction

There has been a major revolution in the field of elective orthopaedic surgery in the past 20 years to the extent that today this field offers the intervention modality most likely to alter radically the life-style of a patient with chronic arthritis. The most important aspect of this topic for the physician is the need to be aware of the importance of patient selection. Results are most gratifying in conditions such as osteoarthritis or adult haemophilia where the patient is well controlled in all respects with the clamant exception of a single surgically accessible joint. In this situation the outlook of the patient may truly be transformed. When, in polyarticular disease such as rheumatoid arthritis, the disease process remains active, advancing and aggressive, caution remains the watchword and the need for sound assessment becomes doubly important.

The only acceptable and realistic surgical goals are relief of intractable pain and improvement in function. Cosmetic benefit is rarely a sufficient indication upon which to rest the case for an operation.

The need for patient education is as important as in any other area of rheumatology and the morale and motivation of the patient are central to success. It must be stressed to the patient that the operation itself is only one part of a complete selection, preparation, operation and rehabilitation programme, albeit a vitally important part. Enthusiastic and skilful pre- and postoperative physiotherapy is of central importance to the final outcome. In no situation is it so important to construct a detailed and comprehensive therapeutic plan involving all members of the team and to check and recheck the progress of the patient towards the therapeutic goal. For example, when multiple surgery is contemplated, a decision on the optimum chronological order will require careful consideration. Attention to hand, wrist and elbow disease may be required before embarking upon lower limb surgery. Flexed knees and metatarsophalangeal subluxation may prejudice the result of otherwise successful hip joint replacement.

If an anaesthetic is required in a patient who might have involvement of the atlantoaxial joints or cervical spine, it is important to X-ray the spine in flexion and extension and to inform the anaesthetist. Hyperextension of the unstable neck may produce paraplegia. Further, temperomandibular involvement may lead to difficulty in intubation.

It hardly needs to be emphasised that any area of skin sepsis precludes surgical intervention until healed. Preoperative weight reduction and control of essential concurrent medication are also obvious points of importance. Patients receiving long-term corticosteroids and diabetic patients require special consideration. The physician may also be involved in decisions such as whether or when to prescribe intraoperative antibiotics or prophylactic low dose subcutaneous heparin.

In general terms the timing of surgical intervention in any single joint is also of critical importance and it is unethical to leave this decision to the "waiting list". Too soon, and conservative measures may not have had a chance to be effective; too late, and rehabilitation may be prejudiced by loss of morale and by the emergence of preventable secondary disease.

In assessing the need for surgery it is important to take into account the degree of success or failure of previous operations and to ask whether or not this may be relevant. Thus it may be possible to avoid altogether the situation where a patient has sought repeated surgery in the past on the basis of wholly unreasonable expectations.

Rehabilitation may be said to begin long before the operation and most certainly becomes more and more important postoperatively. Too often the results of technically successful surgery are abrogated by poor rehabilitation. The most important ingredient in the early days is physiotherapy, but the services of all other members of the health care team may be required in the later stages. Axillary crutches should be avoided in the patient with rheumatoid arthritis, elbow crutches with forearm gutters being more appropriate.

Hand and Wrist

The hand of a patient with rheumatoid arthritis may pose a major challenge to the orthopaedic or plastic surgeon, and too often increasing numbers of operations merely unmask the original failure of assessment.

At the wrist tenosynovectomy and carpal tunnel clearance may relieve the symptoms of otherwise intractable median nerve compression and may prevent rupture of the extensor tendons. Resection of a small amount of the distal end of the ulna may relieve pain and improve grip strength. If too much of the ulna is removed then there is a risk of severe disturbance of hand and wrist joint function. If disease in the wrist is severe, the joint should be arthrodesed in a "cock-up" position. Never perform this operation bilaterally or essential toilet functions become impossible. Flexor tenosynovectomy may release the fixed flexed hand and improve function.

Synovectomy of the small joints of the hand has proved to be most disappointing, but unfortunately so too has replacement arthroplasty of these joints. Whatever the implant chosen, engineering and surgical failure are all too common. Fusion of the joints of the thumb may produce a stable fulcrum and may improve hand function.

Elbow

Synovectomy of the elbow with or without resection of the radial head may produce gratifying early results but later failures become increasingly common. Replacement is still at the research stage.

Shoulder

Surgical options at the shoulder are limited. The problem is inherent in the anatomy of the joint and in its sacrifice of stability in the interests of mobility. Again, replacement remains at the research level and any surgical intervention in the shoulder may leave the patient with a useless upper arm.

Hip

The development of the low friction total hip prosthesis is one of the major surgical triumphs of this century. Success rates in excess of 95% are attained in properly selected patients and mobilisation postoperatively is rapid. This is now the procedure of choice for the irreversibly destroyed hip joint at any age after the epiphysis has fused. The role of synovectomy or arthrodesis has shrunk accordingly, the latter being considered only as a salvage procedure (although even here simple removal of the femoral head alone—the Girdlestone operation—may be preferred).

Loosening and dislocation, either early or at a later stage after operation, or fracture of the bone or the prosthesis may occur, but the most feared complication is infection. This may present immediately postoperatively or may be delayed, sometimes by many years. Interestingly, even in the latter case the infectious agent may have been introduced at the time of the original operation. The frequency of both of these complications has been reduced drastically by a combination of improvement in surgical technique, including the use of laminar air flow theatres, and by the prescription of intraoperative antibiotics on a prophylactic basis. Since many of these patients are elderly, some authorities recommend short-term administration of anticoagulants.

Rarely a syndrome of massive dystrophic calcification around the hip may be seen and the possibility of fat embolus must be remembered both here and in the case of operations around the knee.

Knee

Although at present much less successful an arena, hope springs from the immense amount of research interest centred upon this joint. Again, the problem may be understood easily from an anatomical viewpoint. The knee intrinsically is a much less stable joint than the hip.

Synovectomy of the knee has a much more limited role than in the past and there is no evidence that this procedure protects against subsequent damage. The position in which it may be considered is in the patient, well controlled in all other joints, who has a persistently active proliferative synovitis of one knee without an untoward degree of destruction or fixed deformity. If this has failed to respond to all other general and local measures, including splinting, lavage and the installation of one or at the most two injections of corticosteroid, then it may be reasonable to consider this operation.

Arthrodesis is not an operation which appeals to patients with polyarticular disease since it throws such an immense strain on other joints. Osteotomy may still be indicated in some patients with osteoarthritis.

Constrained prostheses of the Shier's or Guepar variety are seldom used today, their place having been taken by semiconstrained (Attenborough) or unconstrained (Geomedic) designs. In non-constrained models the bone stock should be conserved and bony architecture preserved and the ligaments must be intact. One obvious worry is the possibility that ongoing destructive disease will erode those ligaments, exposing the inherent instability of these prostheses.

Ankles and Feet

Ankle disease is exceptionally difficult to treat surgically. Replacement is still in its infancy and arthrodesis may require prolonged immobilisation to achieve fusion.

Disease of the hind-foot must be differentiated from ankle joint disease. The only movements of the ankle are flexion and extension. Pain on rotation derives from the midtarsal joints. Triple arthrodesis (talo-navicular-calcaneal fusion) may produce gratifying relief in carefully selected cases but may then put considerable strain on the subtalar midtarsal joints.

Involvement of the metatarsophalangeal joints with dorsal subluxation is very common in all of the inflammatory arthritides. The patient complains of a sensation of "walking on pebbles" and mobility may be restricted severely, prejudicing the success of other treatment modalities. The first approach is to try metatarsophalangeal insoles, worn in the correct position, and this is often sufficient. Thereafter the provision of properly fitting and cosmetically acceptable shoes has been made easier by the recent availability of inexpensive lightweight plastics. It is important to stress that up to 4 million pounds sterling are wasted annually in this country by the provision of footwear which is either functionally or cosmetically unacceptable to the patient; this is a scandal! Finally in those few patients who do not respond, excision arthroplasty will produce gratifying results in many instances.

Cervical Spine

In those very few patients with involvement of the joints of the cervical spine in whom there is evidence of advancing neurological symptoms and signs, assessment for cervical spine fusion is required. Both the morbidity and the mortality associated with this operation present formidable obstacles, but on occasion the operation may be life saving.

Conclusion

It can be seen that the role of the surgeon in the management of patients with chronic arthritis is of fundamental importance and may well continue to expand as a result of today's intensive research. It is important that the physician be involved closely if only to ensure the optimum return for the patient.

Subject Index